Hollie d

YOUR BABY, YOUR BIRTH

HYPNOBIRTHING SKILLS
FOR *EVERY* BIRTH

Vermilion
LONDON

1 3 5 7 9 10 8 6 4 2

Vermilion, an imprint of Ebury Publishing,
20 Vauxhall Bridge Road,
London SW1V 2SA

Vermilion is part of the Penguin Random House group
of companies whose addresses can be found at
global.penguinrandomhouse.com

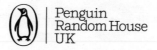

Penguin
Random House
UK

First published by Vermilion in 2018

www.penguin.co.uk

A CIP catalogue record for this book is available from
the British Library

ISBN 9781785041860

Typeset in 8.5/13 pt Futura LT Pro
by Integra Software Services Pvt. Ltd, Pondicherry

Printed and bound in Great Britain by Clays Ltd, Elcograf S.p.A.

Penguin Random House is committed to a sustainable future for
our business, our readers and our planet. This book is made
from Forest Stewardship Council® certified paper.

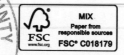

The information in this book has been compiled by way of general guidance in
relation to the specific subjects addressed. It is not a substitute and not to be relied
on for medical, healthcare, pharmaceutical or other professional advice on specific
circumstances and in specific locations. Please consult your GP before changing,
stopping or starting any medical treatment. So far as the author is aware the
information given is correct and up to date as at August 2018. Practice, laws and
regulations all change, and the reader should obtain up to date professional advice
on any such issues. The author and publishers disclaim, as far as the law allows,
any liability arising directly or indirectly from the use, or misuse, of the information
contained in this book.

For Oscar,
I love you more.
It is possible and it is true.

CONTENTS

INTRODUCTION

MY PATH TO HYPNOBIRTHING

If somebody had told me years ago that I would be a hypnobirthing teacher, writing a book about childbirth, I would never have believed them. I had always thought of childbirth as something that women simply had to endure to have a family, and I honestly dreaded the day when I would have to give birth myself. Despite my own mother having had two good births, my only reference was what I'd seen on TV and in films – a dramatic (and often *traumatic*) physical experience. Imagine my angst then, when I found myself unexpectedly pregnant at the age of 25.

At this point in my life I was working for a busy corporate design agency. The environment I worked in was male-dominated and very demanding. I enjoyed my job and I enjoyed my busy life in London. I went out a lot and babies were definitely *not* on my radar.

When I found out I was pregnant – I won't lie – I was terrified. For the first three months (at least) I buried my head in the sand completely, as I think many women do. When you don't yet have a bump it's easy to detach yourself from the idea that there's actually something growing in there – something that you're going to have to get out – and that's definitely what I did until my bump started to show at around four or five months.

Around that time, I decided I should probably start turning my attention towards the birth itself, so I started watching 'horrific birth videos' on YouTube. A word of advice: don't do that.

In hindsight it wasn't a smart move, but at the time it was my way of anticipating a 'worst-case scenario' outcome. I watched these videos through squinted eyes and felt relieved that everyone survived. And that became my goal for birth: survival. If my baby and I were alive at the end of this, I'd consider it a win.

Luckily for me, my partner was a bit older and had lots of friends with children. He seemed much calmer and more positive than me, but I'd put that down to the fact he wasn't about to push a human being out of one of his orifices. He was keen to approach our pregnancy as a team and encouraged me to talk to some of his girlfriends who – in his words – had had 'good' births. I was sceptical, but in an attempt to make him feel involved, I agreed.

When I spoke to his friends and asked them about their births, I couldn't really believe what they were saying. They described their births as 'peaceful, calm, romantic' – not words I had ever associated with birth before. I probed for more information, keen to uncover whatever hallucinogens they'd taken to experience it this way, and it was then that I first encountered the word hypnobirthing.

Now let me say that the second I heard that word I was cynical. *Hypnobirthing*? Giving birth while hypnotised? Pocket watches in the delivery room? Oh god. My first thought was that this was probably not for me, but my partner suggested we book on to a course and find out more. I wasn't massively keen, but I agreed, on the understanding that if we had to sing anything or hold hands with other couples, I was leaving.

So off we went to our first hypnobirthing class; him keen, me cynical (and scared). That was the day my life changed forever.

The thing I found most surprising about the course, right from the off, was that it was largely based on science and logic. We were taught about the female reproductive system and how our muscles were designed to work during the process of birth. This was a revelation to me. I realised I didn't know any of this stuff. Why? How are we not teaching girls about what their bodies do in mainstream education? It's a question you don't really ask until you realise how little you know about your own reproductive kit. And then we learned about the hormones of birth, too. It was enlightening to learn just how capable the system we have in place really is! I learned more about the female body on a 10-hour hypnobirthing course than I had acquired in my whole life up to that point.

And so the shift in my headspace had begun. In just a few weeks I had gone from being terrified about birth to being genuinely excited that I was a strong woman, capable and ready to bring my baby into the world in a calm and empowered way. We'd also begun to really approach the birth as a team. Rather than it being something that I was going to 'do' while my partner looked on helplessly, this was going to be the most intimate and loving experience of both of our lives – and this was a big factor in us deciding we'd like to have our baby at home.

I'm not suggesting you should all have your babies at home, but I'm saying this because I can't emphasise enough how much of a turning point this was in our pregnancy. Rather than viewing birth as an overly medicalised procedure that could only take place in a hospital, we were suddenly talking about birth in a positive way, going to appointments together, practising our breathing, massage and relaxation techniques in the evening, making a playlist for our baby's arrival and generally connecting more as a couple and as parents-to-be. It was the most incredible turnaround.

On Sunday 28 November 2010, my labour began at home. The days that followed were more intimate, euphoric and peaceful than I can do justice to in words. I have never felt so at one with myself as I did during that time. I felt invincible. While the physicality of labour and its sensations were strong and visceral, I can *honestly* say I experienced nothing I could describe as pain. The combination of a snowstorm and my very slow labour meant that we were transferred to hospital after a few days of labouring happily in our little nest, and after an unexpected host of interventions, our son Oscar was born peacefully on Friday 3 December 2010 by emergency caesarean at King's College Hospital in London.

I know what you're thinking, here. She had a caesarean and she's writing a book about hypnobirthing? Yes, I am. Why? Because if it weren't for all the challenges Oscar's birth brought about, I would have had no idea how valuable those hypnobirthing tools really were, and I probably wouldn't be writing this book now. Despite not ending up having my 'dream' birth at home, I was still able to have the most amazing and positive experience – because of hypnobirthing. In fact, I learned even more about hypnobirthing from my son's birth than I had from our course. His birth informed the very essence of my teaching style and the message that I want to get out into the world of birthing women: that a positive birth experience far outweighs a perfect one.

SO WHAT ACTUALLY *IS* HYPNOBIRTHING?

- Hypnobirthing teaches you the physiology of birth: how your body is designed to grow and birth a baby comfortably and efficiently.

- Hypnobirthing teaches you the psychology of birth: how your mind triggers the production of certain hormones during pregnancy, labour and birth, which can either disrupt the natural flow of your physiology or help it work more efficiently. It teaches you how to stay calm during pregnancy.

- Hypnobirthing brings birth back to its primal basics and teaches you how capable the system you already have in place really is.

- Through the use of positive affirmations (which you will see throughout the book) and a sound understanding of the process of birth, hypnobirthing will enable you to clear negative messages around birth from your subconscious mind and re-programme it with beliefs that create calmness and confidence about how your experience unfolds. Rather than gearing your-self up for the trauma and disaster you are inadvertently taught to expect, you will become excited and well equipped for an empowering and enjoyable experience.

- Hypnobirthing values the role of the birth partner, taking them from bystander to knowledgeable, nurturing and supportive asset throughout your pregnancy and on your baby's birth day. You will be encouraged to think and talk about the kind of experience you are trying to create, so that you can work as the best possible team when the time comes. Practical hypnobirthing tools will mean your birth partner can have a tangible impact on how you feel emotionally and how your body responds physically during labour.

- With the knowledge and understanding you gain from hypno-birthing, you will remain an active participant in your baby's birth. You will learn how to ask important questions, how to make informed decisions, how to calmly navigate unexpected turns and how to communicate confidently so that you feel listened to, respected and valued as a mother.

- The wisdom and confidence you gain through hypnobirthing will mean your journey into parenthood will begin as a calm and empowered one. Learning to trust your body, your baby and, of course, your maternal instinct will have a profound impact on your experience as a mother.

- Hypnobirthing isn't a new way of birthing and it requires no leap of faith. Hypnobirthing is allowing birth to happen in a closer alignment to your natural maternal and mammalian instincts. It is birthing with your heart and soul switched on.

The overarching message of this book is that a positive birth experience is more important than a 'perfect' one. So many books about birth promote the idea that the ideal, 'perfect' birth is a natural, drug-free one. But I soon learned (first-hand!) that this is not the reality for so many women. About a quarter of women in the UK will have a caesarean. So before I begin, I want you to know that it doesn't matter how your baby is born! That is not what this book is about. I don't care if you birth in hospital, at home, in a pool, in a car, roaring like a lion or half asleep. I don't care if you have an epidural, a caesarean, or a free birth in the woods: however your baby comes into the world is as unique and special as you are. What I do care about is that you feel fully informed in every decision that you make; that you feel confident in your physical and emotional capabilities; that you trust your birth partner to create and protect a safe environment and to advocate for you; and that you have the knowledge and tools to create an enjoyable, empowering experience where you feel connected with your baby and supported by your caregivers. I care that you are respected and valued at all times and most of all, I want you to realise how absolutely amazing you are.

SOME OF THE BENEFITS OF HYPNOBIRTHING FOR MUM, PARTNER AND BABY

- A mother who understands how her body is designed to work as she grows and births her baby will have the ability to work with it rather than against it. When she understands how her emotional responses affect her physical ones, she can begin practising how to influence them in daily life, as she will then do in labour.

• When a woman feels happy and relaxed during pregnancy, she produces less cortisol – our stressor hormone. While it's very normal to produce a slightly higher level of cortisol when you're pregnant, producing it at a consistently higher-than-normal level can directly affect an unborn child (this hormone passes through the placenta) and can make babies more sensitive to stress when they're born. In fact, consistently elevated cortisol levels have been linked to an increased risk of early miscarriage, reduced foetal growth, and premature birth (associated with a higher risk of the mother developing pre-eclampsia). With the breathing techniques and relaxation tools you'll learn through hypnobirthing, you'll be able to sleep better and enjoy a much calmer, less stressful pregnancy (and have the techniques to help when inevitable stress *does* surface).

• Often in modern western culture, we are very comfortable handing over responsibility for our health and wellbeing to people who we're assured know more than us or are better qualified. While we're obviously lucky to have access to medical support and advances when we need them, it can sometimes mean we slip into what I call 'conveyor-belt' care. Women are treated as numbers or statistics, and that means they're not always getting the bespoke care that is as unique as they and their babies are. With the understanding you'll gain through hypnobirthing, you'll feel confident in asking questions that directly affect you, in making informed decisions that feel right for your family and in seeking out the woman-centred care that will make your experience as personal and empowering as it can be.

- When you understand the process of birth, you will be able to make decisions *with* your caregivers, which means you'll feel more empowered during labour, even if your birth doesn't unfold as you expect it to. However and wherever your baby is born, your experience will always be better when you feel like an active participant rather than a passive bystander.

- This goes for birth partners too. It is such a joy to watch birth partners taking the time to learn about the physical and emotional process of birth so that they know how best to support their partner, not only when the time comes to give birth, but during her pregnancy too. The role of a birth partner is to be by mum's side and on mum's side, and this is infinitely easier when they have taken a keen interest in preparation for birth and beyond.

- Taking time every day to connect with your baby and engage in your practice means that you are getting to know them, and them you. The mother–baby bond starts long before your baby is born, and what a beautiful time this is.

- Believe it or not, unborn babies are very responsive to familiar sounds that happen around them. That's why your baby just wants to be held when they arrive – all they're used to is the sound of your heartbeat and your internal gurgling noises, so it's no surprise that they want to remain as close to that as possible for those feelings of love and security. By listening to your two MP3s (see page 12) on a daily basis, they will become familiar with these sounds and will not only find them comforting during the movement of labour, but also when they are born and in those early weeks and months on planet Earth!

HOW YOU AND YOUR PARTNER CAN USE THIS BOOK

While acknowledging the many amazing benefits of western medicine and appreciating how lucky we are to have access to such fantastic services, my aim is to fill in the gaps in terms of what you can do to make your journey to motherhood a personal and empowering one.

Pregnancy, birth and your experience of life as a woman and a mother are intrinsically linked. One experience affects the other. The more responsibility you take for the decisions you make during your pregnancy, the more empowered your birth will be and the more confident the start of your life as a mother will be. Birth is as much an emotional experience as a physical one, and I want to help you to bring these systems together to function as your most present and powerful self.

Throughout this book, you will find lots of practical information about your pregnancy and the process of birth. You may know some of this already, but one of the key ingredients for a positive birth is feeling fully informed and supported, because let's face it, if you don't know your options, you don't have any. I want this book to reinforce the notion that this is *your* body, *your* baby and *your* birth, and that you are the person responsible for decision-making, every step of the way. Accompanying this information are exercises you can do and techniques to practise – both on your own and with your partner – as well as positive affirmations to take with you on your birthing journey and beyond, as you navigate the world of parenthood.

My advice would be that both you and your birth partner read this book from start to finish. It will give you a sound understanding of the journey you're on, suggestions for things to do together at home and food for thought for areas you want to explore more together. As you read this book, there may be things that you don't connect with right away, and that's okay. Often we have a very set idea about a lot of things, even if we don't have first-hand experience of them, and that's just our subconscious mind trying to be as well equipped for all situations as possible. All I ask is for you to try and approach what I am sharing with you with an open mind. If something doesn't sit right, ask yourself why? Clear your mind and take another look. It is much more beneficial and enriching to form your own opinions and beliefs than to merely adopt those of others. Learning to lean into your intuition and gut feeling will serve you so well in your life as parents and as people of the world. Independent thought is also one of the most valuable gifts you can pass on to your children.

BONUS TRACKS!

Two MP3 tracks (Affirmations and Relaxation) are available with this book, and I advise you listen to them daily if possible from as early on in your pregnancy as you like. The key is listening to them on a daily basis, so even if you don't come across this book until your third trimester, as long as you begin listening to them every day they will still make a difference to your birth. When you go on maternity leave, it can be beneficial to listen to them even more frequently as you get into your mindset for birth. Have Affirmations playing on a loop at home as you go about your daily routine, and try to carve out a rest in your afternoon where you can listen to Relaxation too. These are available at www.penguin.co.uk/YourBabyYourBirth.

The Affirmations MP3 is a series of positive statements about pregnancy and birth. You don't need to be lying down or intently listening to this track, just have it on in the background (it's a great one to have on as you get ready in the morning, or if you're commuting) and these statements will slowly start to penetrate your subconscious mind, which I'll explain about in more detail later (see page 86).

The second track is a Relaxation MP3. Listen to this, if possible, with your partner when you go to bed each night, playing it out loud so that your baby can hear its soothing and familiar tones too. This track is designed to help you relax and fall asleep and will become more effective the more you listen to it.

Listening to these tracks every day means that your mind and body will come to accept them as 'normal'; this means that your mind and body will generate the same relaxing responses when you're in labour as when you have done the practice at home. Believe it or not, many hypnobirthing women will sleep through large chunks of their labour, and this is because they have trained their mind and body to deeply relax throughout pregnancy in preparation for birth.

This daily listening practice is essential if you want hypnobirthing to work, as the effectiveness of these tools is dependent on them being a habitual and familiar part of your routine.

THREE BREATHING TECHNIQUES

As well as listening to these MP3 tracks, I would also like you to practise three powerful breathing techniques on a daily basis. These breathing techniques will facilitate what is happening in the birthing body during labour. Let me explain briefly before I talk about them in more detail later on.

CALM BREATH
A technique that helps quieten your mind at a moment's notice and short-circuit the production of adrenaline in the body. You'll use this breath during moments of stress or anxiety, and also to reset a sense of calm after each surge (contraction). I'll be asking you to practise this breath on a daily basis during any moments of stress, and when you get into bed at night to listen to your Relaxation MP3. (Read how to do this breath on pages 60–61.)

OPEN BREATH
A technique that maximises space in the abdomen to allow your uterus muscle to lift to full capacity, making it easier for your cervix to gradually thin and open. You'll use this breath during a surge in the opening phase of labour. I'll be asking you to practise this breath every morning for five minutes. This will enable you to connect with your baby as you start your day and get a wonderful supply of oxygen

and endorphins flowing around your body before you leap into action. (Read how to do this breath on page 166.)

BIRTH BREATH

A technique that directs energy downwards through your body, helping to engage the muscles of your Natural Expulsive Reflex (NER), which will expel your baby from your body once your cervix is fully open. You'll use this breath during a surge in the birthing phase of labour. I'll be asking you to practise this breath every time you have a poo between now and when your baby's born. This will help you connect with the muscles you'll use when you birth your baby and show you how powerful your breath really is. (Read how to do this breath on page 190.)

TWO PRACTICAL TOOLS

You will also learn two very useful practical tools that help the body to produce endorphins (your body's natural pain-relieving hormones) and oxytocin (the hormone that makes birth work). As a rule of thumb, I would suggest practising one of these two tools every day. Neither need take more than 10 minutes, so it's an easy thing to work into your evening routine with a bit of thought and forward planning.

SOFT STROKING

This is a wonderfully simple massage technique that your birth partner can nurture you with during your pregnancy and labour. The gentle touch of this massage will generate the production of your hard-working birth hormones, while allowing you to slip into a deeply relaxed, cared-for state, switching off your conscious mind and turning your attention inwards to respond to what your baby and body need at a moment's notice. It should be practised at least three times a week for maximum effect. (See page 82.)

FACE RELAXATION SCRIPT

Your birth partner can read this script to you a few times a week throughout your pregnancy and during labour to help soften and open your body in order to make your birth experience as comfortable and efficient as possible. The face and jaw is where we naturally hold most of our tension, which then creates tension in the pelvis, so becoming adept at softening your face will make for a more relaxed and open pelvis when you come to birth your baby. Having your partner read it to you regularly will also mean you begin to associate their voice and particular phrases with a deep state of relaxation. When the mind hears this regularly, it associates it with positive feelings and immediately increases the production of the hormones that make birth easier. (See page 63.)

BIRTH STORIES

Many of the women I have taught have kindly shared their birth stories in this book. With our general dialogue around birth often being rather negative or scary, I believe it to be incredibly important to create a shift by sharing positive first-hand stories of what birth can really be like when you are well informed and have the right tools. As you make your way through these stories, you'll notice how different all the births are and I think that's really important, too.

There are home births, ventouse and forceps deliveries, inductions, hospital births, epidurals and c-sections. I hope this will help you see that hypnobirthing really is for all types of birth. What unites these stories is a thread of women and their birth partners making informed decisions throughout and using the practical tools of hypnobirthing to make their birth better.

KEY TERMS

Throughout this book you will notice that I use language that may be unfamiliar to you to discuss and describe the processes of birth. There is an important reason for this, which we'll explore further on pages 32–3, but for now, a simple explanation is that the language we use affects the way our brain processes information and our experiences. Language is very emotive and, generally speaking, medical jargon can make us feel intimidated or isolated because it has no place in our day-to-day relaxed vocabulary. When it comes to operations and medical procedures, it makes more sense for this language to be used, but in the normal physiological life event that is birth, it is better that we use more everyday language.

I'd like to invite you to start becoming mindful of the language you use when you talk about your pregnancy and the birth of your baby. How you talk about an experience is your choice, so being proactively positive from now is only going to serve you well.

Try not to worry about how your caregivers will react to this more positive language. More midwives than ever are training in hypnobirthing themselves because they are well aware of the positive impact it has on the women they care for, so some of these hypnobirthing terms will be familiar to many caregivers you encounter. Here are the key words and phrases to look out for.

- CONTRACTION becomes SURGE
  The first thoughts that spring to mind when we hear the word contraction is tightening, pain and something that isn't going to be pleasant. Contrast that with the word surge and I think you'll agree that it feels more organic and powerful – almost like a wave of energy.

- PAIN becomes PRESSURE
  Pain is a signal that our body sends to our mind to tell us that something is wrong. When our muscles are getting the blood and oxygen they need during labour (which they will be when you're hypnobirthing), everything works much more comfortably and efficiently. The sensations of labour are much more likely to be experienced as pressure than any pain.

- PATIENT becomes PARENT
  Remember that when you become pregnant there is nothing wrong with you. You are a normal human being who is engaged in a normal life event. As a parent you will use your knowledge and instincts to make the decisions that feel right for you and your family.

- DUE DATE becomes DUE TIME
  In western culture, we have an obsession with charting and dating stuff. We want to schedule things in and label events with time scales and measurements, but pregnancy just doesn't work like that. Every single woman on this planet is different, as is every

unborn baby. We are not robots and every body and every baby works in its own unique way. With this in mind, a normal time for a baby to be born is anywhere between 37 and 42 weeks. That means 37 weeks isn't early, and 42 weeks isn't late. The 40-week estimated due date that we're given in the UK is a date picked in the middle, but the chances of your baby being born on this day are less than five per cent. Thinking of this period as a due time instead takes the pressure off a set day and allows you to feel more relaxed in the run-up to meeting your baby.

- WATERS BREAKING becomes WATERS RELEASING
  I'm not sure something being broken is ever a good thing – and remember this is something that's actually *meant* to happen in labour. With that in mind, we talk about our waters releasing instead of breaking.

- COMPLICATIONS become SPECIAL CIRCUMSTANCES
  Sometimes birth does not unfold in the way we envisage, but that doesn't mean it can't be a positive and empowering experience. This book is very much designed to help you have a positive birth experience rather than obsess over a perfect one – it doesn't exist! Rather than thinking of unexpected turns as complications, which automatically makes things sound difficult, we think of them as special circumstances. Your ability to make informed decisions calmly and confidently will mean you are able to navigate these turns with ease.

ENJOY YOUR JOURNEY

I'll wrap up here by wishing you the very best for the rest of your pregnancy and while working your way through this book and the world of hypnobirthing. Know that you are a very strong and capable individual who is well equipped to have a really wonderful birth experience. Learning how your body works and teaching your mind to work with it rather than against it will transform your baby's birth and make your first profound experience as a mother a joyful one that you will want to remember forever. Let your birth partner support and advocate for you and let them nurture you so that you can nurture your baby. Make a commitment to your practice and give this stage of your life the weight of importance it deserves. The more work you put into this and the more responsibility you take for your own wellbeing, the better your birth will be. It really is that simple. Birth is safe and you are strong.

I am preparing for the
birth of a calm baby and
a confident mother.

HONEY'S BIRTH
SHARED BY FEARNE COTTON

My two pregnancies were VERY different. I won't go into too much detail about my birth with Rex, yet know that he came flying into the world with a suction cup on his head and a lot of long limbs flaying around. It wasn't that calm and I didn't feel prepared. It goes without saying though that I feel beyond blessed that I have this incredible little chappy in my life, and feel proud and elated that my little cone head (temporarily) screamed his way into the world on a snowy night.

My birth with Honey was very different. Mainly because I tried a different route. I heard about the wonderful Hollie de Cruz through a friend who had experienced a very calm and joyful birth not long after my first. I was intrigued and slightly unbelieving of the whole anecdote so immediately got in touch. After meeting with Hollie and learning some integral breathing techniques and visualisations I felt slightly more prepared packing my hospital bag and slightly less nervous when that first contraction began. The fear and expectation had been completely replaced with pure excitement. It was already working.

I opted for a water birth this time round as I had heard wonderful things about delivering in the water. This isn't always an option if you have complications or if there isn't a pool available at your local hospital but I struck gold as it seemed not many other babies were wanting to come into the world that particular morning. I slipped into the water and instantly felt more at ease. As the surges grew in intensity so did my mental strength. I pulled all available visualisations and mantras from my arsenal and surfed through each wave of intensity knowing I was going to be OK. This was all so new and so different from my previous experience.

After a few hours of this cyclic rollercoaster I flipped over, without thought, on to my hands and knees. It was almost an animalistic urge. I could feel Honey moving downwards and each time she shifted my mouth let out an another-wordly howl. Not of pain but of strength, release and power. I felt wild, empowered and very connected to everything around me. A small baby with a shock of red hair floated out into the water around me. My beautiful ginger angel didn't make a noise. She was calm, unfazed and serene in her presence as I picked her up for the first time. Even writing this now the whole episode seems completely dreamlike and surreal.

I learned the power of breath, how your body and mind can very much work in tandem, and that no two births are ever the same.

PART ONE
PREGNANCY

Congratulations on your pregnancy! Whether you have only just found out that you're expecting or have come across this book in the last days of your pregnancy, the techniques of hypnobirthing that you will read about in these upcoming pages will help make your birth a better experience. In the past, hypnobirthing has received a bit of bad rep because it sounds much weirder than it actually is. Yes, when I first stumbled across it I thought there would definitely be pocket watches involved, but in fact, it's all really quite simple, and based upon the science of being a woman.

Since time began, female mammals – humans included – have been giving birth. This process is designed to work. Its intricate physical system and deep emotional wiring are part of us and are intended to operate harmoniously. Hypnobirthing isn't just about the birth itself though, it's about understanding who you are and how you work; it's about taking back the reins of your own health and wellbeing; and it's about nurturing yourself throughout pregnancy and into your life as a mother.

The techniques I'll be sharing with you are designed not only to improve how you feel during your pregnancy but will help you bond with your baby. Hypnobirthing also helps you to connect with your birth partner in a profound and intimate way as you prepare for this new chapter as The Ultimate Team. And even if you don't have a partner on this journey with you, you will be taught how to train your mind and your body to respond to your cues and enjoy reaching new depths of calmness and confidence whenever you need it. As you begin to take more responsibility for the care you receive, you will become competent in asking questions and confident in making informed decisions that feel right for you and your baby, even if that means going against the status quo.

During your pregnancy, your intention should be to prioritise yourself and give specific time and thought to growing your baby, rather than living mindlessly alongside it. Yes, we have a physical system in place that takes care of the science of growing a baby, but what we so often overlook in our busy western lives is the profound effect that your emotional experience of pregnancy has on the development of your child, the bond you'll share and your experience of motherhood. Many of us have this notion that 'pregnancy won't change me'. But that mindset will only inhibit you from experiencing the emotional depths that this sacred time offers up. I urge you to be courageous enough to put yourself first. Put your baby first. Worry less about what others might think and more about your own wellbeing, even if this has not been a habit in your life so far.

I'll go into more details about how to care for yourself later on, but my first request of you is to be ready to learn how to sleep. It sounds simple, but it amazes me how many people function on so little sleep and think it's something to be proud of. Sleep is really important to all of us but even more so during pregnancy. Our body does all of its essential repair and restorative work when we're sleeping, so it's imperative for both you and your baby that you are getting a good-quality sleep every night. Of course, I know that's easier said than done during pregnancy, when you're going to the toilet more frequently or are kept awake with restless legs! Using my daily Relaxation MP3 (see page 12) will ensure that you are slowly drifting into a deep sleep without the distractions of looking at your phone or watching TV before bed. Make sure you're listening to it every single night whenever possible, and your body will begin to associate it with the relaxation you'll want to access in labour. Tools like this will benefit you now, during the birth of your baby and definitely when your little one is here and sleep becomes even more precious!

Surround yourself only with positive messages of birth. Stop watching reality TV shows about giving birth and if a well-meaning friend starts reeling off their traumatic birth story, politely ask if you can pick up the conversation once you've had your own experience. We'll talk about this more as we go along, but something I'll be inviting you to do is to release any embedded fears you may have acquired about birth from your subconscious mind. We're going to be reprogramming this part of our brain with positive messages about birth, and you can make a head start on that by beginning to listen to your Affirmations MP3 (see page 12). Play it at least once a day, every day – maybe on your commute or even just have it on in the background as you get ready in the morning or cook or bathe in the evening.

The exercises I'll set as we go along are important and designed to fit into your life. Take them seriously and commit to them but, most importantly, keep an open mind as we go along. Birth can be so much better than you think. Believe me.

Where my mind leads, my body will follow.

CHAPTER 1
OWNING YOUR PREGNANCY

YOUR BODY, YOUR BIRTH

Something fascinating I've observed in my time as a birth educator, is how seemingly willing women are to hand over the reins of their experience to someone else – normally a medical professional. I am by no means suggesting that these people can't be an amazing asset to a positive birth experience and a source of great comfort and wisdom throughout your pregnancy, but it is absolutely essential that you realise that *you* are the person that will make the biggest difference to the journey you and your baby are on. Birth is a normal, physiological process that women (and all female mammals for that matter) have been nailing since time began. As a woman, your body is designed to birth a baby – you were built for it and you have been preparing for it physically and hormonally for years, even if not consciously.

Think about it: for any other significant life event – job interview, holiday, wedding – we spend time planning and preparing. You wouldn't go along to your driving test having never had a lesson behind the wheel, even if you knew where the brake and accelerator were. You'd spend hours, weeks and months learning the rules of the road, hazard awareness, and the ins and outs of how to get from A to B safely and confidently. It's a cliché I know, but knowledge really is power. As is practice. If you learn a new language, you can read a book about it or take classes, but it's the time you put in to practising your knowledge – to actually speaking the language – that gives you confidence in your ability, and that ultimately makes your experience of using this new language an easier one. It may sound strange at first, but this is all true of birth too.

Getting ready for birth, learning about the process and practising how you will breathe, think and feel during birth is what hypnobirthing is all about. The skills and techniques you learn during pregnancy will help you feel prepared and confident for birth and well equipped for your journey as a mother. If you want a positive birth, you need to prepare for one. It's time to face any fears and dispel them, through knowledge and also with easy ways to bring yourself back to a place of calm emotion and physical ease.

WORKING AS A TEAM

It's also important to know that you are not alone. Yes, you'll ultimately be the one birthing your baby, but know that there is a wonderful team of people around you who are there to help you at every stage. You will no doubt have already met with midwives and/or doctors, you may have a group of local pregnant friends who you meet up with and discuss all the details of your pregnant body, or you may have a network of close family members to support you. But on the actual day, it's your birth partner who will be your voice when you need them, who will support you and who will help give you energy when you need it. Get them involved as soon as possible during your pregnancy so that they can be part of the whole journey. They, too, will then be better informed of what you may need.

⌐   ⌐

When you trust that your birth partner is able to communicate on your behalf, you have the best chance of a calm, comfortable and efficient birth.

L   ⌐

Birth partners – and dads, in particular – can often feel like a bit of a spare part. Because appointments and then the birth itself usually happen in a hospital, birth partners often think that they're the least knowledgeable person in the room. In truth, they are likely to know mum better than anyone else, making them an absolute expert in what she's going to need. Whoever your birth partner is – your partner, a close friend or a relative – there are lots of things that he or she can do to help. Ultimately their role is to protect and advocate for you, so that you feel safe and able to relax – and that starts now.

TALK
Discuss with your birth partner the kind of birth experience you want to create and be open to re-evaluating this as your pregnancy progresses. When you first found out you were pregnant, you might have felt that a home birth was THE ONLY THING you wanted, or maybe you were set on giving birth in the swankiest hospital with doctors at every

corner – but that doesn't mean you can't change your mind. The more you work together and communicate clearly on a regular basis, the more trust and intimacy you will build up to take into the day of your baby's birth and beyond. And of course, the more able your birth partner will be to be your advocate for you – communicating with caregivers will, after all, be one of their most important jobs.

QUESTIONS TO CONSIDER WITH YOUR BIRTH PARTNER:
- How will they communicate with caregivers in a way that allows you to remain in a quiet, relaxed state when you don't feel like interacting yourself? Will they take conversations outside of the room for instance, or will you want to be there?

- How can they help you to relax if they see you getting anxious? Is there a favourite song they could play that can be your trigger for happiness? Can they put a hand on your shoulder to reassure you that you're safe? Is there a favourite affirmation they could recite?

- How can they make your environment as comforting as possible? Do you want lights off or very dim? Would you like some music to be playing? If you get too hot, would a cold flannel be more suitable than being fanned (I personally found the latter rather irritating during labour!)?

- What would you want to happen in the event of special circumstances arising? If you needed to be in theatre for instance, should your birth partner stay with you or start skin-to-skin contact with your baby?

- How can your birth partner look after you in the postnatal period? Could they bring you food? Arrange for a postnatal reflexology appointment or massage? Get a stock of ideas built up so that they can support you in the best possible way after birth and as you navigate those early days and weeks.

ATTEND ANTENATAL APPOINTMENTS TOGETHER

This immediately aligns you together as a team. It also means that your birth partner is well informed, so that during birth you can switch off from your conscious mind – the one that responds to questions and asks them – allowing you to turn inwards and respond to your body in an intuitive and primal way.

CREATE A CALMING ENVIRONMENT

We will talk later about ways you can create a calming environment for birth but get into the habit now of spending time together in a relaxed and stress-free space. By doing this you will both learn what it is that brings you back to a state of calm; by practising feeling calm, you can take these skills with you into birth. If your partner feels calm and confident they will also bring this reassuring energy into the room – and what a wonderful thing that is! Explore ways in which your partner can help create a calm, safe environment.

Ideas might include:
- Dimming the lights
- Diffusing essential oils
- Helping create a birth playlist
- Soft stroking massage (see page 82)
- Applying pressure to your back where necessary
- Reading the face relaxation script (see pages 63–5)
- Playing the Relaxation and Affirmations MP3s (see page 12)

BOND WITH YOUR BABY TOGETHER

I think it comes quite naturally to lots of mums to talk to their bump or give it reassuring pats and strokes throughout the day, but this can feel like more of an alien activity for dads and birth partners. The good news is, babies aren't bothered about the quality of your chat – just hearing your and your partner's voices will become very reassuring for them. They're obviously going to hear mum's voice all the time, meaning it will become very familiar, but by practising the face relaxation script and even by just having your regular conversations about this new adventure, your baby will hear your partner's voice in a calm and loving way, and will no doubt recognise these comforting tones when they are born.

> # My birth partner is by my side and on my side.

POSITIVE LANGUAGE

The subconscious mind is like your own personal hard drive. Acting like a sponge, it is very sensitive to language and will generate reactions based on the feelings it has stored for certain words. If someone shouted 'get down' or 'run', it is very likely that you would do so without asking for a rational explanation. Language is very emotive and has the power to impact how we experience the world around us, so it is essential that we use it mindfully. This is also fundamental in how you approach your pregnancy and another big step in assuming responsibility for the birth experience you want to create.

So, let's look at the traditional language of birth. Think about how the word 'contraction' makes you feel, or what it makes you think of. Don't think about it too much, just be aware, in this moment, of the first couple of words that spring to mind. Now do the same now for the word 'surge' – what feelings does that bring about for you?

I think you'll agree that surge generates more positive feelings of power and energy, whereas contraction brings about images of pain and tightening. It's clinical, rather than natural, as is so much of the dialogue around pregnancy and birth. I fully understand that you may be reading this thinking that using the word surge instead of contraction is not going to have any effect on what you experience, but I promise you it will. We expect a contraction to be painful, but we can set new, more positive feelings for the word surge.

Think about more of the language of birth, such as waters breaking. If something's broken it usually needs to be fixed! Try waters 'releasing' instead; for pain, try 'pressure', 'energy' or 'waves'. When we change the way we talk about birth, our subconscious mind helps us to experience it differently. Be mindful of the language you use from here onwards, and familiarise yourself with the terms you'll find in the introduction on page 17.

Speak positively and ask those around you to do the same. If people start talking to you about pain, politely ask them to choose their words more thoughtfully.

FLORES'S BIRTH
SHARED BY ANOUSHKA PALAVATHANAN

Even though people around me seemed desperate to label my labour as 'traumatic', I can hand on heart say my labour was the most amazing, intense and positively challenging experience of my life. Two and a half years later I can remember birthing Flores like it was yesterday, and it was beautiful.

But it was no walk in the park. Although the journey did actually start with a massive walk in the park. I got the classic pre-labour surge of energy and just felt I had to get out of the house and go on a two-hour hike on my own. At nine months pregnant. Wise!

I got home, sat on the sofa and felt my waters break. It was just a little trickle, no massive movie gush, so I spent 10 minutes convincing myself I had just pissed my pants. Luckily, better judgement took hold of me and I called my home birth midwife who confirmed there was vernix present so things were starting.

I was having surges at this point but they weren't very strong, just that familiar tightening and hardening feeling over my tummy. Because my waters had gone the midwives told me I had 24 hours to get into active labour or I would need to be induced due to the risk of infection.

This is where the hypnobirthing really came into its own. As a self-confessed control freak the deadline could have really sent me into a spin, but Pali and I just breathed through every surge, got into the fresh air and let the process unfold before us.

But by Wednesday (Pali did some heavy-duty midwife negotiations to keep me at home for 72 hours) my surges were still on and off, so we headed into hospital for an induction. Bye-bye lovely hypnobirth nest of candles, music and looking into my husband's eyes; hello manic labour ward, medical professionals and lots of distractions.

But as soon as we got to our bay, Pali took over, closed the blinds, put on my headphones, got the lavender going and told everyone who came into contact with me that we were doing hypnobirthing. And so the nest came with us and it was surprisingly easy to dive back into the 'zone'.

I was examined and told I hadn't dilated at all, even though I was 2cm dilated on Tuesday evening. Feeling demoralised I was induced. I had no access to water (no pool, no shower, not even a hot water bottle for health and safety reasons!). We were drifting further and further from our birth plan. So we leant on everything we had learned and just focused on each other, the breathing, the affirmations and the light touch massage.

The surges came pretty quick and hard after that but at 2am I was examined again and told I still hadn't dilated. So, again, we refocused and dug really deep together. I was given gas and air but it made me sick. So I went through the night of increasingly strong surges on breathing and Pali's support.

By 9am on Thursday morning the surges were so strong I asked for an epidural. I was tired after several days of stop/starts and it just felt like the right thing to do in the moment. We were transferred to our own room at last, which Pali quickly made our own, with fairy lights, affirmations on the wall and music playing.

My midwife (who I hadn't met before) was absolutely incredible. She examined me and I was 7cm! I had gone from zero to 7cm in seven hours on hypnobirthing techniques alone, I felt like Wonder Woman! Then the epidural kicked in, which meant I could sleep for the first time in 36 hours, while my body continued to surge.

By 7pm on Thursday I was 10cm dilated and ready to bear down. We agreed to let the epidural wear off so I could connect with the urge to push. I remember this stage of labour so vividly. I was assured that this phase took 30 minutes to one hour max. Four hours later she still wasn't coming out. We could see her hair but she was stuck with her face to the side. I was running out of steam. The consultant was called and I was told that I needed to get to surgery for either suction, forceps or caesarean delivery. I had been fully dilated for so long the medics were worried about bleeding after the birth. So at 11.30pm on Thursday night I had my first ever experience of theatre. With our music playing and my contact lenses out I still felt totally serene and in control. After a failed attempt with the suction cup the consultant explained that forceps were the last option before a caesarean. I was determined to birth her vaginally after the journey we'd been on. So when a surge came I pushed with every bit of energy I had.

And there she was, born at 12.03am on 5 June. On my chest, covered in vernix and looking like an old Peruvian man: Flores, the best thing that ever happened to us.

HYPNOBIRTHING YOUR WAY:
EXERCISE 1

Now have a go at exploring your own thoughts and feelings about birth. In your journal or just on a plain piece of paper, draw a cloud and fill it with words that you want to represent your birth experience. How do you want to feel? What words make you feel safe and at ease? Keep this piece of paper close and look at it often. Stick it on the wall wherever you decide to have your baby and focus on the words that bring you strength and peace. You can even do the same for motherhood and keep it with you in the days, months and years to come.

I speak positively,
I think positively.

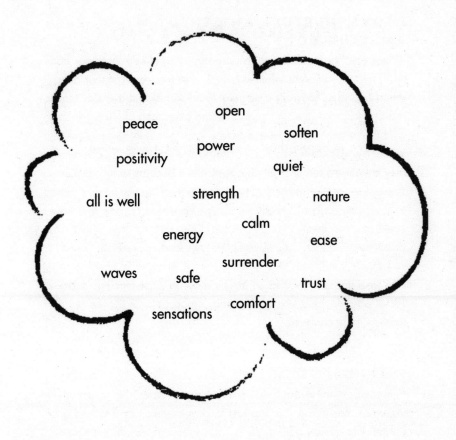

open
peace
soften
power
positivity
quiet
strength
all is well
nature
calm
energy
ease
surrender
waves
safe
trust
comfort
sensations

I LOVE, NURTURE AND ENJOY MY AMAZING BODY

When you first find out you're pregnant, it's unlikely that your body will look any different when you look in the mirror, but that doesn't mean how you *feel* isn't changing dramatically. I remember feeling really disconnected from my body at the beginning of my pregnancy, as if it was being taken over by some force of nature (which I guess it was!). My skin went crazy and I broke out in spots, my boobs felt like they weighed a ton and became so tender, I became super sensitive to smells and went off all of my favourite foods. However, when I started learning more about exactly what was happening inside and how I could nurture these changes rather than distract from them, that disconnect soon turned into complete awe and admiration.

Let's take a closer look at what you may be experiencing, and find some ways to help you understand, embrace and nurture yourself through these changes.

1. FATIGUE

I remember being so tired in my first trimester that I genuinely thought I was dying. I'm not just talking having to go to bed a bit earlier, but literally getting up to make a cup of tea and then having to have a lie down because I felt so depleted. This kind of fatigue is completely normal during pregnancy because your body is working so hard, especially during the first trimester while it grows a placenta to look after your baby's needs and to cope with the physical and chemical changes that your pregnant body demands.

TOP TIPS TO COPE WITH FATIGUE:

- Go to bed earlier

  Of course you want an evening with your partner when you get in from work but try to just bring everything forward a little bit. Prepare food that doesn't take hours to cook, or batch cook at weekends so that you can eat earlier during the week. Sleep quality is much better before midnight, so securing an extra hour before midnight will make a big difference to how you feel the following day.

- Create a bedtime routine

  Unwinding before you fall into bed will mean you drift into a deeper sleep more easily, rather than lying awake wishing you could just switch off. Run yourself a warm bath (or ask your partner to do this for you), light some candles, listen to your Affirmations MP3 (see page 12) and use a relaxing essential oil such as lavender. Diffuse this in your bedroom too or use a pillow spray, and then get into bed and listen to your Relaxation MP3 (see page 12) rather than watching TV or scrolling through your phone. You will enter into a deep sleep now that you've slowed yourself down and let your mind quieten.

- Enforce a digital detox

  It's so tempting to get into bed and start scrolling like a pro. This is not the time. Set a household rule (yep, that means your partner has to adhere to it too!) of no screens for 15 minutes before you get into bed. A time frame like that makes it manageable and the benefits you'll start to feel of a quieter mind will give this little ritual longevity.

- Exercise

  It might feel like the last thing on your mind if you're exhausted, but exercise can actually improve the quality of sleep you get, meaning you don't feel so tired the following day. It's advisable to consult your caregiver about the types of exercise that are safe for you and your baby during pregnancy, but finding something like a pregnancy yoga class or even simply incorporating more walking into your day can really help you to adapt to growing a human, while maximising the benefits of more energy and better sleep. I remember joining a pregnancy yoga class and finding it really reassuring just to be around other pregnant women, especially as I was the first in my group of friends to be expecting.

2. MORNING SICKNESS

Okay, so this is no one's idea of fun. Although it can be totally miserable, remember that this is the manifestation of your body and hormones adapting to pregnancy. It's also your first opportunity to start listening to your body and responding to its needs – a skill that will prove invaluable as the weeks and months go by. Remember also that it is likely to lessen (or hopefully disappear!) after the first 12 weeks or so. If you've just found out that you're pregnant and you're feeling a bit ropey, be proactive and start implementing some of these natural remedies to make those first few months as comfortable as possible.

PLEASE NOTE: SOME WOMEN DO EXPERIENCE SEVERE MORNING SICKNESS, HYPEREMESIS GRAVIDARUM (HD), WHICH DOES REQUIRE SPECIALIST TREATMENT.

TOP TIPS TO COPE WITH NAUSEA:

- Magnesium

  This clever mineral helps balance cortisol, our stress hormone. But during pregnancy, our hormones can sometimes inhibit the proper absorption of magnesium. Excess cortisol can cause us to feel sick and tired, and when combined with our pregnancy hormones this can leave us feeling doubly nauseous and exhausted. Try a magnesium spray rubbed into your skin, morning and evening, or add magnesium flakes to a bath or foot soak and turn it into an opportunity to nurture your busy body and relax! Adding magnesium flakes to the bath as part of your new bedtime routine (see page 41) and listening to your Affirmations MP3 (see page 12) while you soak is a lovely way to incorporate this practice into your day.

- Travel bands

  Not just for motion-sick coach-trip fanatics! They work using acupressure points on the wrist. Simply pop a band on each wrist with the button placed face downwards over the Nei Kuan, an acupressure point that is located between the two wrist tendons, three finger widths from the wrist crease.

- Peppermint and lemon

  Peppermint has a calming and numbing effect that instantly relaxes your stomach muscles. Drink it as a tea (fresh leaves or as a teabag) or use the essential oil: burning or diffusing it around the house, adding a few drops to a bath or inhaling from a handkerchief that you keep with you throughout the day. Lemon is an effective alternative – a good tip I came across was to keep lemon wedges cut up in the freezer to nibble on whenever nausea calls.

- Ginger
  You've probably thought about drinking it in tea form (handy to keep at work and as a replacement for caffeine) or nibbling a ginger biscuit, but my favourite is to keep some candied ginger in your handbag. Not only will it help keep your blood sugar levels up when you may not feel like eating much, but it tastes delicious and feels like a bit of a treat!

- Calm breathing
  The calm breathing technique that I will introduce you to on pages 60–61 is a brilliant remedy for feelings of nausea. Often when we start feeling sick, we begin to panic at the thought of being sick and this just makes everything worse. The next time you feel nauseous, try taking a few moments to acknowledge that your body is working hard and reward it with a few minutes of calm breathing to relax the mind and soften the body.

3. BREAKOUTS AND BLOATING

If you're tired all the time and you're feeling sick, chances are a skin breakout, along with bloating, constipation and wind, are the last things you need. However, these are all very normal things to expect in the first trimester of pregnancy. The change in hormones can also make your skin seem extra oily, so if the acne from your teenage years suddenly reappears, don't be alarmed!

TOP TIPS TO COPE WITH CHANGES IN YOUR SKIN:

- Water, water, water

  Hydration during pregnancy will not only help with feelings of fatigue but it will also help service your skin during the hormonal changes that are going on behind the scenes. If you find it difficult to drink enough water, set little anchors for yourself throughout the day. For example, every time you check your phone, have a sip of water too. You could even recite a little affirmation in your head as you drink; something like 'I listen to my body and respond to its needs'.

- Prioritise self-care

  Because your skin changes so much during pregnancy, it's a really nice idea to treat yourself to a new skincare product that will help you feel nurtured. If your current skincare routine is aggravating your skin, don't feel like you have to stick with it! Step into the new and embrace your different requirements. Also take time in the evenings to look after your skin properly. Maybe get your partner to rub some oil into your belly, and then you can take off your make-up while tuning into your breathing. The more you can combine breathing with other activities, the easier it will be to do in labour!

HYPNOBIRTHING YOUR WAY:
EXERCISE 2

Are there other symptoms that you're suffering with right now? If so, get a piece of paper and pen and write down the symptom. Think about what it feels like physically and how it is affecting you emotionally.

Next (without looking it up on the internet!), think about why this symptom is manifesting and what it could mean your body is doing or trying to do. Whatever that is, write it as a positive statement.

Finally, I want you to imagine that a close friend has written to you saying they are suffering with this symptom, and I then want you to 'write back to them' with some advice. What should they do to look after themselves? How can they alleviate the stress that this symptom is bringing, or make it easier to live alongside? How can they put themselves first and look after themselves in light of what they're experiencing? See the example on the next page.

SYMPTOM:

I'm feeling really forgetful and absent-minded.

PHYSICAL MANIFESTATION:

Feeling groggy and tense, sometimes with a headache
or light-headedness.

EMOTIONAL MANIFESTATION:

Feeling frustrated with myself at not remembering things
and feeling anxious that I'm losing part of my brain!

WHAT'S MY BODY TRYING TO DO?

Balance my hormones and also access a different, more
subconscious part of my psyche, because growing a baby requires
different tools to my usual everyday activities.

MY POSITIVE STATEMENT:

My body and mind are working hard to prepare me for becoming
a mother, and it's okay if other bits of my mind take a break while
I process new experiences.

ADVICE TO A FRIEND IN THIS PREDICAMENT:

Be kind to yourself. Keep a little list of things you need to remember
so that you don't feel so much pressure to keep on top of it all in your
brain. People love you and will understand if you have other things on
your mind. Prioritise your sleep and do lots of relaxation practice so
that your mind and body are getting the rest they need.

Give it a try! I bet you find it therapeutic, and this is a brilliant activity
that you can keep revisiting as your pregnancy progresses and how
you feel continues to change.

PREPARING YOUR BODY FOR BIRTH

Although much of hypnobirthing is concerned with getting yourself into a good mental state ahead of the birth, we all know that the body and mind are intrinsically linked. A healthy body supports a healthy mind and as part of your preparation, you should aim to get your body ready for birth too. Be mindful of what you eat and drink and how you exercise, knowing that you are making choices for your baby as well as for you. (Although baby will probably enjoy the odd chocolate biscuit too ...) Try and take a proactive approach to your wellbeing and recognise the effect that this will have on your long-term physical and emotional health. Looking after yourself now will put you in the best position for a great birth and a healthy start to motherhood. When we combine eating well, exercising, good-quality sleep and teaching the mind how to quieten, we think more clearly and feel more energised in everyday life. This is the beginning of taking responsibility for your baby and your birth.

GOOD NUTRITION

In those early weeks and months, when morning sickness is likely to be at its peak, you may find that all your efforts to eat well go out the window as you exist on a diet of baked potatoes and candied ginger (see page 44). But as soon as you feel able, try to get your diet back on track so that you absorb as many vitamins, nutrients and minerals as possible – as well as fibre. Your body does require additional nutrition as it adapts to pregnancy and growing your baby but the idea of 'eating for two' is a bit of a myth. Poor eating habits and excess weight gain over the next few months may also increase the risk of a condition called gestational diabetes, which can potentially lead to pregnancy or birth complications, so part of taking responsibility for your birth means being mindful of what you're putting into your body in the run-up.

Some of the key ingredients and food groups you should be aiming to include in your diet and why:

- Dairy products
  These are a great source of protein and calcium, both of which help support the needs of your developing baby. Dairy provides high amounts of B vitamins, phosphorus, magnesium and zinc. If you're not a big milk drinker, then Greek yoghurt is a good way to incorporate this food group into your diet.

- Eggs
  A good source of protein, fat, vitamins and minerals. They are also a good source of choline, which is a vital nutrient that will support the healthy development of your baby's brain and spinal cord. Just make sure they are stamped with the British Red Lion quality mark, which drastically reduces any salmonella risk.

- Fruit and vegetables
  These are a really important part of a healthy diet because of the numerous vitamins and minerals they contain. Vitamin C is really important for immune function and also helps the body to absorb iron. Oranges, berries and bell peppers are a good source of vitamin C and will also help boost your water intake. Vitamin A is another important vitamin needed as your baby develops. One of the best vegetable sources of this is sweet potato.

- Vitamin B9 (folate)
  This is something that many of us don't consume enough of, so you may have been advised to take folic acid, which is folate in synthetic form, prior to conception and during your first trimester. This is fine, but by incorporating foods like lentils, peas, beans and chickpeas into your diet you can access folate in a natural way. In fact, one cup of lentils provides 60–90 per cent of the recommended daily allowance of folate.

- Dark and leafy greens
  Greens like broccoli, kale and spinach are not only rich in antioxidants, but offer another good natural source of calcium, iron and folate and also contain vitamins C, K and A. If you find yourself suffering from constipation during pregnancy (or afterwards!) the high fibre content in greens like this will help.

- Dried fruit
  Prunes and dates are another good remedy for constipation. High in fibre, potassium and vitamin K, dates are even said to encourage a natural start to labour as you approach your due time. It's worth bearing in mind that dried fruit does contain a lot of sugar, but opting for non-candied versions and sticking to one portion a day makes for a good snack and healthy dose of important nutrients.

- Avocados
  A good source of fatty acids, which are important for the growth and development of your baby. They are also high in fibre, folate, potassium, and vitamins K, C and E. Potassium can also help relieve leg cramps and restless legs, which so many pregnant women suffer with.

- Whole grains
  These include brown rice, quinoa, buckwheat, oats and bulgur wheat. Many women crave bland, beige food in the first trimester, but opting for whole grains over refined grains like white rice, white bread, white pasta and products made with white flour will mean that you're benefiting from the fibre, B vitamins and magnesium they contain. Oats also contain a good amount of protein, which is particularly helpful if you're not feeling like eating as much meat during pregnancy.

- Omega-3 and vitamin D
  Both have an important role to play in the development of the brain and eyes of a developing foetus, and fish such as salmon, mackerel, trout, kippers, sardines and cod are rich in these essential fatty acids. While you want to be mindful of your mercury intake during pregnancy, eating two portions of oily fish each week should mean you're consuming an optimal amount of omega-3. Salmon is also one of the few natural sources of vitamin D, another tricky one to get enough of in normal diets. Vitamin D boosts bone strength and helps to build a healthy immune system. There are also links between low vitamin D levels and an increased risk of pre-eclampsia, so it's worth taking seriously. If you don't eat fish or seafood, you can use fish liver oil as an alternative source of vitamin D, although this shouldn't exceed one tablespoon per day. (This is not to be confused with cod liver oil, which should be avoided due to its retinol content, which in concentrated doses could harm your unborn baby.)

STAY HYDRATED
Your blood volume increases during pregnancy, making it even more important to stay hydrated. If you find yourself suffering from

headaches, fatigue and the kind of patchy memory that's often labelled as 'baby brain', it may be a sign that you're dehydrated. Drinking around two litres of water a day will also help prevent UTIs and constipation, to which you are naturally more susceptible during pregnancy.

PREPARE YOUR BIRTHING MUSCLES

The perineum is the area between the vagina and anus. If you start massaging this from around 34 weeks for about five minutes each day, it can increase muscle and tissue elasticity to make a vaginal birth more comfortable. You can do perineal massage by yourself, but it can also be an intimate massage to share with or have done by your partner. Here's how to do it:

1. Find a comfortable position, using pillows to support you and keeping your legs bent at the knees to better reach the perineum.

2. Use a vegetable-based oil (I'd recommend almond oil) and apply to the fingers and thumbs, as well as the entrance to the vagina.

3. Place your thumbs inside your vagina and then press them firmly towards the anus and against the sides of your vagina until you feel a tingling sensation. Massage this area in a U-shaped motion, starting for just a minute at a time, and working up to five minutes as and when you become more comfortable with it.

Another way to prepare your pelvis for birth is to regularly exercise your pelvic floor. There are lots of different techniques to strengthen this area, but the most common is to simply sit comfortably and

A GUIDE TO PERINEAL MASSAGE

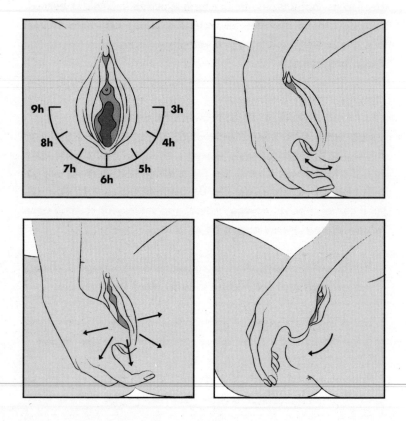

squeeze the muscles (as if you were stopping urination mid-stream) 10–15 times in a row. Try not to engage your abdominals or bum or thighs or hold your breath while doing this. Hold each squeeze for a few seconds before releasing and repeating.

There is now a brilliant product on the market in the UK and Ireland called an EPI-NO. This innovative birth training device can be used from any time during the pregnancy to exercise the pelvic floor muscles, but from 37 weeks the exercises also enhance the function of the natural pregnancy hormone relaxin. It prepares the perineum with gentle stretching exercises, which reduces the risk of tearing or the need for an episiotomy during birth, so in essence, it covers the job of the two things we've just talked about. I know lots of women who have used this and rave about it; find out more about it at www.epi-no.co.uk.

I listen to my body and
I do what it needs me to do.

SAM AND HOLLY'S BIRTHS
SHARED BY LOUISE TRAVIS

My husband and I stumbled across hypnobirthing when we were researching alternatives for pain relief, as my options were limited due to previous surgery. It wasn't well known at the time and I remember when we spoke to our friends and family about what we were doing, they looked at us with a mixture of amusement and bewilderment.

Hollie and hypnobirthing supported us through the birth of both our children. They were quite different births, but both were (dare I say it) amazing!

Our son, Sam, was born in hospital in water; both he and I were calm and relaxed throughout. The midwife and student midwife who helped deliver him both commented that they hadn't seen a birth like it (and one of them had been a midwife for 12 years). I don't think I was particularly amazing, I just think we were so incredibly prepared for birth and so in control due to all the work we did with Hollie.

Second time around, due to the amazing positive experience we'd had delivering Sam, we opted for home water birth. Our daughter, Holly, arrived slightly quicker into the world – so quick in fact that my husband didn't have time to blow up the birthing pool! But while it was a different and quicker experience, we once again felt in total control and confident in her delivery.

Hollie and hypnobirthing had an incredible influence on our experience of birth, so much so that our daughter's name is in no small part due to Hollie!

The best way I can describe hypnobirthing is that it gives you (and your partner) the confidence that you can deliver your baby. By being confident, it enabled us to stay in control and relaxed throughout, which in turn led to a drug- and intervention-free delivery for both our children.

I could write an essay about the birth of our children and the experience, but in summary I don't care how many people thought we were slightly mad and New Age to be doing hypnobirthing – IT WORKS!

RELAX . . .

In the early days of your pregnancy, it can be easy to forget all the hard work your body is doing, especially as you won't necessarily look pregnant yet. Add to the mix that you probably haven't told many people your news, it's tempting to just carry on as normal, but that can be at the cost of your emotional and physical wellbeing. If you're pushing yourself too hard, your stress hormone (cortisol) will spike, which also leads to increased feelings of nausea and fatigue, and generally not feeling like 'yourself'.

One of the best things you can do to combat this is to really listen and respond to your body's needs. This means getting lots of rest whenever you can (think early nights and weekend naps!). Also get into the habit of using a relaxation aid such as my Relaxation MP3 (see page 12). This will help you to relax, physically and mentally to a very deep level, leading to a reduction in cortisol and an enhanced feeling of wellness.

Ultimately, it's important to remember that your body is working really hard right now, and it's essential that you listen and respond to its important messages. You're going to need to do this for the rest of your pregnancy – and into motherhood – so it's good to get practising now. Culturally we are obsessed with *doing*, and it's important to remember that sometimes there's just as much value in *not*.

Getting yourself into a relaxed state is one of the key lessons of hypnobirthing. When you are relaxed, you allow yourself to give birth. Your journey with hypnobirthing is all about getting as adept as possible at relaxing quickly, even in stressful situations. The more familiar you become with listening to your body when you are deeply relaxed now, the easier it will be when you are experiencing the sensations of labour.

Practise relaxing as much as possible: in the bath, in bed, on the Tube, at work, in the car, walking in the park. Practise tuning in with your breath and releasing tension from your body and it will become a completely normal and rewarding response for you to draw on when you bring your baby into the world.

THE SYMPATHETIC AND PARASYMPATHETIC NERVOUS SYSTEM – OR WHAT HYPNOBIRTHING ESSENTIALLY BOILS DOWN TO

There are two parts to the body's nervous system: the sympathetic nervous system and the parasympathetic nervous system. It sounds complicated, but in actual fact they are just long names for two different primal responses within the body.

THE SYMPATHETIC NERVOUS SYSTEM

The sympathetic nervous system is our emergency response unit – a life-saving reaction that triggers the fight, flight or freeze mechanisms. When we feel afraid, the body releases catecholamine and adrenaline to usher us to safer surroundings.

THE PARASYMPATHETIC NERVOUS SYSTEM

The parasympathetic nervous system is at the opposite end of the spectrum. It is active during our normal, calm state. It promotes oxytocin production in the body, which we know is the hormone that aids labour and birth (see page 148).

The most important point to remember about our sympathetic and parasympathetic systems is that they cannot function at the same time: we are either feeling relaxed, safe and calm OR fearful and anxious, but we cannot experience both of these together. The key to a calm and comfortable birth is to remain in a parasympathetic state throughout birth, so it's important to learn how we can achieve this.

LEARNING TO RELAX

When we talk about relaxing, we often think of doing something we find relaxing, like watching TV, cooking or socialising with friends. While these things really can be relaxing, it is quite far from relaxation in its truest form. When we relax wholly and deeply, our body functions in its parasympathetic state and is able to produce more endorphins. We are able to meet our inner selves and, ultimately, experience feelings of peace and safety.

If you're anything like me, you'll find it incredibly hard to switch off at a time when there are so many changes afoot. I remember doing pregnancy yoga when I was expecting Oscar, and I'd spend the whole class thinking about what I still needed to buy, when I would finish work, which socks to pack in my hospital bag, and so on. I don't think I'd ever really actively 'relaxed' before and learning how to do it properly changed my life. I think people have the misconception that switching off is too hard, so rather than worrying about *switching off*, think of it as *switching in*. I'm going to show you just how easy it is to do this by introducing you to our first breathing technique and then giving you a guided relaxation exercise for you and your partner to practise at home.

CALM BREATH

This calming breath is very simple and once it becomes established it will enable you to relax at a moment's notice. You will use it after a surge during labour but you can practise it during pregnancy in any moments of stress. Try it when you get into bed at night to listen to your Relaxation MP3, or when your birth partner reads you the face relaxation script on page 63. This is a breath we will come back to time and again so keep practising it until it is familiar to you, as that is when it will become most effective.

1. Stop what you're doing and sit comfortably.
2. If you're in a sitting position, place your feet flat on the floor.
3. Soften the posture of your jaw and shoulders.
4. Breathe in through your nose to a slow count of four.
5. Breathe out through your nose to a slow count of six.

Repeat this breath while you visualise inhaling peace and exhaling tension. When I was in labour, I found it helpful to actually visualise these words (peace and tension), but experiment with what feels most natural to you. You could try inhaling while visualising a white light and exhaling a blue light (or whatever colours take your fancy) or imagine the waves of the sea lapping in with your inhale and out with your exhale. There really is no right or wrong way to visualise this breathing technique; just find what feels right for you and do that every time so that it begins to become instinctive. Some people even like saying the count to themselves in their head, and that's fine too.

HYPNOBIRTHING YOUR WAY:

EXERCISE 3

Practise this breathing technique – the Calm Breath – whenever you feel any kind of anxiety or tension creeping into your system. Maybe it's someone cutting you up in traffic or when you get an unpleasant email at work. At times when your natural response would be to feel on edge or agitated, draw upon your calm breathing technique to short-circuit that stressor response and replace it with feelings of peace and ease.

I'd also like you to practise it whenever you do the face relaxation script (see page 63) or the soft stroking massage on page 82. In labour, this breath is going to be useful in moments of tension and also after each surge has subsided to quieten your mind and reset a sense of relaxation throughout your body.

FACE RELAXATION SCRIPT

Many of us hold tension in our head and face without even realising. When I used to work in an office, I remember wondering why I had such a stiff neck, shoulders and bad head every day. It was because I was staring at a screen not breathing properly and holding all of this pent-up energy in the top of my body. Notice how your body feels right now. Are your shoulders soft? Is your jaw relaxed? Are you frowning or does your forehead feel at ease? Becoming more aware of these areas physically will serve you so well in labour, because tension in the face and jaw creates tension in the pelvis. The more relaxed your face is, the softer and more open your pelvis will be – and this is obviously good news on your baby's birth day.

Your partner can help by reading this script to you during your pregnancy. The more they do this for you, the more effective it will be during labour. It will help promote complete relaxation in your mind and muscles, which will get those all-important endorphins flowing and your birth system relaxed. It's also a lovely way for your baby to hear your partner's voice in a gentle and loving way. We know that babies are incredibly responsive to sound from inside the womb and they will become familiar with your partner's voice the more they hear it. There's nothing more beautiful to see than a baby moving its eyes in the direction of voices it recognises when they're born. It's pure magic.

I really hope you enjoy having a go at this one, but if at first you find it hard to follow or to relax to, don't worry. Remember that this is a brand new skill you're learning, and sometimes it just takes a bit of time. The more you practise this exercise, the easier it will become for your mind and body to respond to the anchors of relaxation and the more enjoyable and instinctive it will become. Don't worry either if you laugh! It's very likely that you haven't heard your partner read in a soft, slow voice before, so it's bound to generate some giggles. We produce loads of endorphins when we laugh, so this is a brilliant response too. Essentially, as long as your partner doesn't *scare* you by reading this script, you're winning!

FOR PARTNERS TO READ ALOUD TO YOU

(Note to partners: you don't need to put on a new voice for this. Chances are that mum loves your voice, so just be yourself but read more slowly and softly than you usually would. Use lots of pauses to give mum time to action your suggestions and prompts, and don't be afraid to tweak the language or add/remove bits that make it sound more 'you'.)

Make yourself comfortable and begin to focus your attention inwards to the rise and fall of your breathing and just close your eyes. Don't force them shut, don't hold them shut. Just allow them to gently meet and feel how comfortable it is to just allow your eyes to remain gently closed.

Now place your awareness on your breathing. Breathe fully and breathe easily. Let your breath flow all the way down through your chest and your stomach. Let it drift all the way down to the soles of your feet.

As you feel the relaxation drifting throughout your body, become aware of how heavy the muscles in and around your eyelids are becoming. Feel all the little worry lines begin to smooth out and relax. Your eyelids are now closing more thoroughly. It almost seems as though they are sealed.

And now they feel as though they are locked shut. You know you could open them, but as you try it seems to be too difficult for you to open your eyes. They feel so comfortable.

Now just imagine that same deep relaxation drifting down over your cheeks and your jaws. Your face and your jaw set the pace for the rest of your body and you now feel your shoulders begin to feel relaxed and limp, beginning to sink into the frame of your body. Feel your elbows becoming limp and relaxed – all tension drifting away. With every breath you relax more and more.

In a moment, I'm going to count from 1 up to 5. When I reach 5 you'll open your eyes and return to your surroundings, feeling mentally alert, physically energised and emotionally calm and confident.

1 – Tuning back in with your breathing. Inhaling peace, exhaling tension.

2 – Hands and fingers beginning to move.

3 – Feet and toes beginning to move.

4 – Eyelids feeling lighter.

5 – Wide awake and feeling great.

(Note to partners: When you use this in labour, leave out the parts where you count mum back out of relaxation. You can leave mum to relax or sleep. Maybe continue the relaxation with some soft stroking or by putting on your birth playlist.)

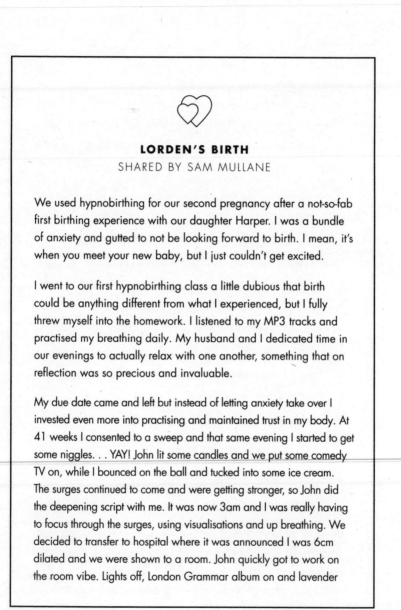

LORDEN'S BIRTH
SHARED BY SAM MULLANE

We used hypnobirthing for our second pregnancy after a not-so-fab first birthing experience with our daughter Harper. I was a bundle of anxiety and gutted to not be looking forward to birth. I mean, it's when you meet your new baby, but I just couldn't get excited.

I went to our first hypnobirthing class a little dubious that birth could be anything different from what I experienced, but I fully threw myself into the homework. I listened to my MP3 tracks and practised my breathing daily. My husband and I dedicated time in our evenings to actually relax with one another, something that on reflection was so precious and invaluable.

My due date came and left but instead of letting anxiety take over I invested even more into practising and maintained trust in my body. At 41 weeks I consented to a sweep and that same evening I started to get some niggles. . . YAY! John lit some candles and we put some comedy TV on, while I bounced on the ball and tucked into some ice cream. The surges continued to come and were getting stronger, so John did the deepening script with me. It was now 3am and I was really having to focus through the surges, using visualisations and up breathing. We decided to transfer to hospital where it was announced I was 6cm dilated and we were shown to a room. John quickly got to work on the room vibe. Lights off, London Grammar album on and lavender wafted under my nose. The light touch massage was my saviour, which surprised me massively as I imagined touch would annoy me. At the beginning of each surge I would simply grunt 'touch me', directing John to stroke my leg or arm! This was unbelievably effective; I found it relaxing, comforting and it really did ease the surges. Prior to labour I had written all my positive affirmations on Post It notes, so I stuck my favourite ones to my thigh to help maintain focus during the surges. I visualised ocean waves through a lot of the surges and I was surprised to be nodding off in-between many of them.

At about 7.30am my waters went with what felt like a pop followed by a gush. It was an amazing feeling of relief but then almost instantly I got the urge to push. The pressure of the surges had gone and it was just this strong wave that took over and directed my body with what to do next. I found this the most amazing and empowering feeling. I was then, and still am, amazed at the female body – or more importantly my body!

I felt the baby's head with my hand in between a pushing surge and this was when the midwife stated, 'the baby is completely back to back – it's not often you see them coming out looking at you. You're amazing to be doing this with just gas and air!'. With a super feeling of self-pride, I breathed our boy out . . . all 9lb 7oz of him with a head full of hair and huge eyes staring up at me! The placenta followed fairly quickly afterwards with the support of the midwife. I couldn't believe I had done it, and we had a boy! I am still amazed at how different it was compared to my first birth, all thanks to hypnobirthing. Hypnobirthing gave me such strength and guidance to hold on to in moments of doubt or worry.

Relaxing my mind relaxes my muscles.

HELP YOUR BABY GET INTO THE OPTIMAL POSITION

The best *physical* prep for birth is through exercise, eating well and posture. Poor posture, from our mostly sedentary lifestyle, can cause tension and twists in the pelvis, which aren't particularly helpful in getting our babies into the best position for birth. The position of your baby can have a big impact on what happens in birth, so it is something to be mindful of throughout your pregnancy.

Here are some ways you can help baby into an ideal position for a comfortable birth:

- If you sit at a desk at work, replace your office chair with a birth ball, at least for some of the day. This will put less upwards pressure on your pelvis and allow more space for your pelvis to relax.

- Another tip for the workplace is taking in a footstool to rest your feet on under your desk. Not only can this keep your pelvis balanced, but it can stop your feet and ankles feeling so swollen at the end of the day too!

- Take regular breaks from sitting to stand up and walk around. Tie it in with other things you know are important, like getting up for a drink of water or regular snacks. Stretch your legs and use a couple of calm breaths to open up your abdomen and clear any tension from your mind.

- Take up some gentle exercise like walking, swimming or pregnancy yoga. These activities encourage gentle movement in the hips and pelvis, which will help create more room for your baby to get down into a great position.

- In the evenings, sit on a birth ball (or lean over it) if you're watching TV. Slumping back on a sofa closes up your pelvis and makes it harder for your baby to move into an optimal position for birth.

- Consider investing in a pregnancy pillow (a bit like a long soft sausage!) for when you sleep. These will help you to sleep on your side more comfortably, especially if you have a tendency to roll on to your back during the night – and they make a great breastfeeding cushion too!

BABY POSITIONS IN WOMB

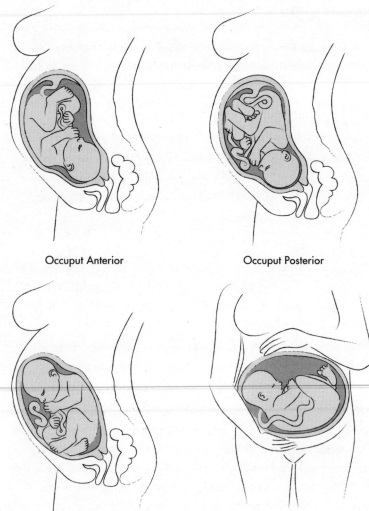

Occuput Anterior

Occuput Posterior

Breech

Transverse

OCCIPUT ANTERIOR (OA)

This is considered the ideal position for your baby to be in, where your baby is head down and facing your back. In this position, your baby will have their chin tucked towards their chest, meaning that the smallest part of the head meets the cervix first.

OCCIPUT POSTERIOR (OP)

In this position your baby is head down but facing your front – it is often referred to as 'back to back', meaning the baby's back is against yours. During labour, some babies will actually rotate into the OA position as the uterus muscles surge.

TRANSVERSE

A transverse baby lies across the womb in a sideways position, with their head to one of mum's sides and the bottom across her other. This is very normal up to 26 weeks, but a transverse baby at full term will need to be born by planned caesarean section.

BREECH

A breech baby is bottom down with head towards the top of mum's abdomen. If your baby is in the breech position and is born vaginally, the bottom will normally be born first (which is called 'frank'), but in some cases the feet and bottom can arrive together ('complete') or they arrive feet first ('footling'). Only 3–4 per cent of babies are in the breech position at full term, but to give you an idea of how normal it is for babies to turn before that time, 25 per cent are breech before 28 weeks. If your baby is breech by 36–37 weeks, you should be given the choice of a natural breech birth or a planned caesarean section. Speak to your healthcare provider about your options.

Always consider that whichever position your baby is in, it might be in the right position *for them* but if at 34 weeks your baby isn't OA, you are likely to be offered the option to have them 'turned'. This is called ECV (external cephalic version). You do not have to agree to this if you don't want to, and alternative therapies such as osteopathy, acupuncture, moxibustion (see page 75), reflexology and chiropractic care can be very effective in loosening the ligaments or adjusting the sacrum to allow the baby to adopt a head-down position more readily. Whatever you decide, make sure you are fully informed and speak to your healthcare provider about your options.

ALTERNATIVE THERAPIES

Most of us in the developed world are used to turning to western medicine when we encounter any health-related problems. But with the effects of clinical drugs on a developing baby still questionable, many women during their pregnancy look for alternatives to modern medicine to help the body heal and thrive.

Over my time as a birth educator, I have spent a great deal of time looking at how birth is approached in other parts of the world. One thing that has always struck me, is how in less-developed communities – where birth is no-frills in terms of medical input – the care of a woman becomes much more nurturing and holistic during her pregnancy. Women are often massaged or bathed a lot during pregnancy or take part in other nurturing rituals. As simple as this sounds here in writing, its effects shouldn't be underestimated. We know that when a woman feels relaxed and safe, she functions in her parasympathetic nervous system, where her body produces the hormones she needs for birth to unfold comfortably and efficiently (see page 152). When she is stressed, anxious and tired, the opposite happens and the process of birth can be a lot more difficult. Now, these parts of the nervous system shouldn't be thought of as something we start controlling only when we go into labour, but rather something we begin exercising as early as possible.

For the best birth experience, it is crucial that we start preparing the body for the physicality of birth during pregnancy. Alternative therapies are often thought of as an indulgence or merely a way to 'pamper' ourselves, but seriously ladies, stop thinking of looking after yourself as a treat! Nurturing your body results in nurturing your baby and it will help set you up with the best start to your journey as a mother. Rather than leaving the outcome down to luck, I urge you to start prioritising your own wellbeing as an essential part of pregnancy.

I consider alternative therapies to be a regular part of my physical and emotional health maintenance. If I'm not sleeping properly, rather than taking sleeping pills as a quick fix I'll look for the root of the problem and nurture it holistically so that it stops happening. As a result, I have become so much more in tune with my body and empowered in my own health. By learning a little about the treatments available and by incorporating them into your pregnancy and beyond, you can do the same.

Although alternative therapies don't need to replace the conventional antenatal care you'll receive during your pregnancy, they can offer a brilliant way to relax and tune into how your body is changing.

Of course, if you do decide to explore these therapies further, it is important to consult your GP or midwife first and to find a fully qualified and insured practitioner who can work with pregnant women.

ACUPUNCTURE

Acupuncture is the practice of inserting very fine needles into your skin at key points on your body. They are believed to act on the meridian (energy) lines that run around your body and can be used both as a preventative measure and to help ease certain symptoms and conditions.

Here is acupuncturist Claire DaBreo on how regular treatments can benefit you during pregnancy:

A comfortable, healthy pregnancy is something every mother-to-be would like and acupuncture can be a safe and effective way to address all manner of pregnancy-related conditions, from sciatica and pubic symphysis dysfunction (caused by misalignment in the pelvis) to heartburn, morning sickness, fatigue, depression, carpal tunnel syndrome and more.

Pre-birth acupuncture, undertaken from 36 weeks, is a series of weekly treatments that specifically prepare the body for birth, and practitioners have a dual approach. The first is focused on promoting a natural, efficient labour by using a set of points that help prepare a woman's body for birth, with an emphasis on affecting the cervix and pelvis and promoting the optimal position of the baby. The second aim of treatment at this time is to address the 'minor' issues many pregnant women are dealing with at this stage: heartburn, fatigue, anxiety, constipation, swelling, difficulty in sleeping, for example, are all commonly reported. While not in any way life threatening, they can make the final weeks of pregnancy that bit more uncomfortable.

Finding a practitioner with specialist postgraduate training is strongly recommended and local ACT (Acupuncture Childbirth Team) groups are a good place to start, though they aren't active in all parts of the UK.

Moxibustion (another traditional Chinese therapy involving burning dried mugwort on the body) is often used in conjunction with acupuncture. It is believed to help turn breech babies (see page 70) and should be done as near to 34 weeks as possible.

REFLEXOLOGY

Reflexology is based on the theory that different points and areas on the feet, lower legs and hands correspond with different areas of the body. Key benefits include relaxation, renewed mood, tension release and improved sleep and general wellbeing.

Reflexologist Hannah Adams shares her experience:

My midwife suggested I try reflexology when I was approaching 42 weeks pregnant with my first child. After treatment I wished I had invested in regular sessions throughout my whole pregnancy. I later decided to retrain as a reflexologist, inspired by the potent simplicity of the therapy.

Because the benefits of reflexology are cumulative, it is recommended that sessions start sooner rather than later. Treatments can be taken in the first trimester although some women prefer to wait until after 13 weeks' gestation. Fortnightly or monthly appointments are then recommended, increasing to weekly sessions post 37 weeks, in preparation for labour.

It is commonly thought that reflexologists can 'induce' labour. We can't, because induction is a medical procedure. What we can help to create, however, is the optimum calm, relaxed and supported environment for natural labour to begin. The effects of deep relaxation on an anxious mum's mind, muscles and nervous system can't be underestimated as she awaits the birth of her baby. Visualisation, breathing techniques and sharing any worries within the safe space of a reflexology session can also help women leave the couch feeling lighter, brighter and more empowered.

OSTEOPATHY

Osteopathy is based on the principle that the structure of the body influences the way it functions. It can be effective in the treatment of symptoms such as musculoskeletal pain, including muscles, tendons, ligaments and joints, headaches, digestive and circulatory issues, and an inability to relax. Many women consult osteopaths for pain relief during pregnancy and osteopaths receive many referrals and recommendations from midwives and others involved in the care of pregnant women.

Osteopath Nancy Nunn adds:

While pregnancy is a state of health rather than an illness, the profound changes that take place through these nine months require the pregnant mother's posture to make significant adjustments. During this time, the chemistry of her body changes too, as the balance of hormones is altered. One of the major effects of this change happens within the musculoskeletal system. In preparation for accommodating her expanding uterus and growing baby, as well as the anticipated process of labour, ligaments and other structures become much more stretchy. This creates greater flexibility in her pelvis in order to aid passage of her baby through the birth canal. These changes have other beneficial effects too: women who had overly stiff spines prior to their pregnancy may find that their discomfort eases during pregnancy. However, greater flexibility in the ligaments also means that it is easier for some women to overstretch their joints. In this case, osteopathy can be used to relieve pain and restore function.

A pregnant mother's posture also changes as she accommodates her growing baby. The slowly increasing weight of her uterus and its contents means that the position of her spine and associated muscle tone need to change to maintain her balance around the body's centre of gravity. This usually causes her normal spinal curves to increase, requiring flexibility in each joint. Previous unresolved injuries are common reasons why a pregnant mother's posture struggles to effect this change, often causing problems from the middle of the second trimester onwards as her baby's rate of growth increases. In this case, osteopathy includes a full assessment to identify not only the structures causing her pain but also any other mechanical features preventing postural adaptation.

Some pregnant mothers visit osteopaths in the last trimester in order to encourage their baby to achieve an optimal intrauterine position (see page 70) and prepare their body for birth. Her spine, pelvis, ribs and abdominal wall provide the 'container' in which the growing baby, uterus and placenta reside alongside her other organs. Tight muscles and joint strains can compromise this space and lead to awkward positioning for the mother and for the baby in her uterus. White osteopaths do not directly move the baby, they seek to create a more relaxed and comfortable space, which encourages the baby to adopt a more favourable position.

Some osteopaths choose to pursue specialised postgraduate training in the care of an expectant mother. Osteopaths are also able to suggest exercises to help to relieve pain and restore function. Mothers may also seek help from osteopaths after the delivery to address the effects of the delivery on their own bodies as well as their baby.

CHIROPRACTIC

Chiropractic care is a wonderful therapy that identifies and treats misalignments of the joints and spinal column, which can cause physical discomfort by affecting the nerves, muscles and organs.

Doctor of Chiropractic, MaryAnne Shiozawa is a specialist in pregnancy chiropractic adjustments. She explains:

There are many factors that can help you experience a healthy, happy pregnancy. Most of them you already know: diet, exercise, sleep, rest and reduced stress. Body work, such as pregnancy chiropractic care, is another great way to help prepare your body for pregnancy and birth.

Many women who have experienced pre-existing back problems find their symptoms become exacerbated as their body changes during pregnancy. It is also common for women who were previously unaware of any issues in their spines to suddenly experience lower back and pelvic pain during pregnancy, as the baby gets bigger and ligaments get laxer (more bendy and stretchy). Instability is another huge issue for some women, and it can lead to a stressful pregnancy with lack of movement and constraint for you and your baby.

I recommend regular weekly chiropractic care sessions that should ideally start pre-conception, as it is also believed it can help prepare the body for conception. After conception, chiropractic care should continue weekly to check for common first-trimester discomforts such as nausea, fatigue and cramping. Regular chiropractic care for hyperemesis (severe morning sickness) can improve or lessen the severity and duration of symptoms.

As your spine and pelvis change each week to accommodate your growing baby, embedded tension in your body can sometimes cause areas to become 'stuck' along the nerves, joints, muscles and ligaments. Other areas may over-compensate for these areas of 'stuckness'. Regular chiropractic adjustments will allow for your brain and nervous system to naturally connect and communicate to all the necessary areas to release that tension.

Studies show that regular chiropractic care from pre-conception to birth, as well as postnatally, has huge benefits for both mother and baby. It is taking a proactive approach, helping the function and alignment of your whole system before issues arise, rather *than waiting and seeking 'damage control'. Women find their pregnancy is more comfortable, that they have more energy and experience better restful sleep, less heartburn and fewer general aches and pains. It has also been reported that women undergoing chiropractic care during the third trimester go on to have shorter and less painful labours, with smoother progression and with fewer interventions, such as an epidural or assisted births, including c-sections.*

Many women seek chiropractic care for the Webster Technique, in which I am certified, to help the alignment of the pelvis and uterus to allow for the baby to find its ideal birthing position. Many women whose babies are breech find their babies reposition themselves after having a series of Webster Technique pregnancy adjustments.

In my clinical experience, pregnant women love receiving chiro-practic care, especially those who have noticed a huge change from having painful pelvic problems to enjoyable comfortable pregnancies and births. Check out www.icpa4kids.org and www. shiozawawellness.com for more information on pregnancy and chiropractic care.

MASSAGE

Massage in pregnancy is usually a combination of remedial massage, shiatsu and acupressure. The treatment takes place in a side lying position with your bump, knees and ankles fully supported and is a wonderful support physically and mentally during pregnancy, labour and the postnatal period.

Pre- and postnatal massage therapist Beccy Hands explains the benefits:

Pregnancy massage doesn't have to mean an hour of gentle stroking – your body can take a good old pummel if your therapist is trained properly as we know how to get right into those tight spots safely and effectively. Let's face it, there's nothing worse than a massage therapist stroking over an unhappy muscle, it's just a tease! So, what are the benefits of pregnancy massage?

There are SO many!

Firstly relaxation. This can help with so many pregnancy related ailments: nausea, hormone imbalances, stress and anxiety. Need another excuse for a guilt-free massage? The endorphins you release during massage actually cross the placenta, meaning that baby gets the relaxed, blissed out feeling too! Everyone's a winner!

Massage can support muscles that are working harder, so in turn can ease backache, pelvic pain, hip and leg tension and discomfort. We can work with restless legs, calf cramps, SPD, sacroiliac tension, sciatica and sore necks and shoulders to name just a few discomforts associated with pregnancy.

Massage provides 'time out' for mum to be, to enjoy bonding with the growing bump and feeling looked after – growing a baby IS tiring and a bit of TLC does you the world of good. Finally, massage most often will result in a fantastic night's sleep, as the body is brought back into balance. This can be a very welcome side effect later on when sleep patterns can become a bit more erratic.

SOFT STROKING MASSAGE

The soft stroking massage technique is a wonderful way for your partner to nurture you during pregnancy and labour. The more this simple technique is practised, the more readily your body will respond to its endorphin-inducing effects when you need it most.

1. Help mum find a comfortable position which gives access to her back. An easy and comfortable one to try at first is to face a wall with your hands pressed against it at head height. Have your feet hip width apart (or a little wider if more comfortable) and remain upright and leaning forward.

2. Imagine that the back is like the map of a tree. Mum's spine is the trunk, so think of lots of branches coming out of the trunk and going all the way up the back and over her shoulders.

3. Starting at the bottom of the tree (the base of mum's spine), use the back of your fingertips to softly trace the pattern of the first branches, both left and right at the same time. Go all the way out to mum's sides. At the sides, remove your hands and come back into the trunk, ready to climb the next branches.

4. Continue slowly and gradually all the way up the tree until you reach mum's neck. At this point, you can go up the neck and into the scalp using the same soft stroking technique.

5. Be sure not to drag your hands over mum's back or use too much pressure, as the skin can be extra sensitive during pregnancy and a rubbing sensation can prove irritating. By using a very light touch, you are stimulating nerve endings on mum's skin which help her body

produce endorphins – her body's natural pain relief – and promote physical comfort and relaxation. To gauge your pressure, if you were touching any more gently, you wouldn't be touching at all – it's that light!

A few points about the soft stroking technique:

- Mum may find the sensation ticklish and that's okay! That shivery flinch is a sign that her body is responding brilliantly to your touch.

- Practise this in different positions and on different parts of the body. You could do it on the inside of mum's arm while you're both watching TV, in the palm of her hand or over her neck and face. You could even stroke her bump as a lovely way to bond with your baby at the same time. Practising in different positions and scenarios will mean the technique is more easily applicable in labour. For instance, if mum is in a comfortable position in labour but you can't access her back, you'll need to adapt and improvise, so try and do this at home so that it's easier in labour.

- Make sure you find a comfortable position too! Some women like a lot of this stroking in labour, so it's really important that you find a position you can offer it in. Again, practice makes perfect!

- Don't worry if mum doesn't seem like a massive fan right now, but keep up the practice. I couldn't see myself enjoying this in labour AT ALL when I was pregnant, but it was my saviour during a long labour and I'm so glad we'd continued to practise it or I know we wouldn't have used it.

- This technique can be used postnatally too. If mum's feeling fractious or finding breastfeeding uncomfortable, give her five minutes of the soft stroking massage just before a feed so that her body starts producing those feel-good and relaxing endorphins.

- You can even use this technique on your baby to help ease discomfort or calm them when upset or agitated. Do it in exactly the same way on their back while holding them over your arm. They love it!

Each day I nurture myself so that I can nurture my baby.

BUZZ'S BIRTH
SHARED BY GIOVANNA FLETCHER

I hadn't heard of hypnobirthing until I fell pregnant with Buzz, and I had no idea what Hollie would be doing with us when we started our course. Fast forward 11 weeks and it was time for Buzz to make an appearance – almost three weeks ahead of schedule. Even though I was sat in a restaurant with a table of friends when my waters broke, I felt extremely calm about the whole thing. In fact, I stayed and finished my steak even though my friends wanted to shout out for towels or call an ambulance. I knew none of that was necessary; I had time, and I was happy. That was all that mattered.

That said, we left the table before pudding (the only time that's happened in my life) and started heading home. We rang the hospital and, seeing as we were passing anyway, they said to stop by. Nothing was happening, they said. I'd either wet myself (which is fairly common in late pregnancy) or it was my fore waters. I was sent home. But I couldn't sleep because my surges were coming so often, so I sat in the dark on my big pregnancy ball, while listening to Coldplay. It was so peaceful.

A few hours later my doctor called. He was going away that night and wanted to check me over before he left. 'Have you been having contractions?' he asked, clearly perplexed. 'I'm having one right now.' The look of shock on his face still makes me chuckle now.

I was 6cm dilated, so he felt it was the right time to head to the hospital. Seeing as I hadn't eaten in a while, we decided to make a detour and have brunch. I think that was the only part of the day where I questioned my sanity. The afternoon was filled with light touch massages, listening to calming scripts or Coldplay, and chuckling along to Michael McIntyre on the television.

When my son was handed to me for the first time, I told the midwife that I'd just had one of the most amazing experiences of my life. I stand by that statement. Labour, birthing, breathing – whatever you want to call it (I've never been too fussed about the terminology side of things) – was the most powerful adventure I'd ever witnessed my body go through.

Our bodies are pretty awesome – and our minds, extraordinary.

AFFIRMATIONS

Positive affirmations are a great way to make positive language part of your everyday life. You will find lots of them throughout this book. Some will resonate with you more than others, so choose those that have meaning for you. With your partner – or even with a pregnant pal – write down your favourites on to some sticky notes and place them around your home in places where you'll see them regularly between now and when your baby arrives. Every time you see one at home, I want you to stop, smile and say it out loud. You may feel a bit strange doing this at first, but it's a great way to make positive language part of your daily routine and let these good messages penetrate and embed in your subconscious mind. Also see pages 32–3 for more on the power of positive language.

HYPNOBIRTHING YOUR WAY:
EXERCISE 4

1. Think of something you struggle with – perhaps a habit, mindset or belief.
2. Write it down as a single sentence.
3. Now rewrite its positive equivalent.

For example:
1. Making time to practise.
2. I find it hard to make time to practise my hypnobirthing techniques.
3. I make my hypnobirthing practice a priority because I intend to have a great birth experience.

Now you try!

Every time you become stuck on something or struggle to overcome a habit or thought process, come back to this exercise and create positive affirmations that are as unique as you are. Keep hold of them all over the course of your pregnancy so you can look back on how far you've come in shifting your mindset from negative to positive. This will give you a great boost and that extra confidence for labour.

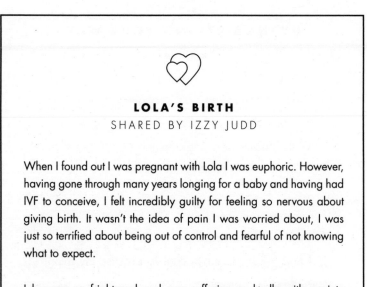

LOLA'S BIRTH
SHARED BY IZZY JUDD

When I found out I was pregnant with Lola I was euphoric. However, having gone through many years longing for a baby and having had IVF to conceive, I felt incredibly guilty for feeling so nervous about giving birth. It wasn't the idea of pain I was worried about, I was just so terrified about being out of control and fearful of not knowing what to expect.

I became so frightened and was suffering so badly with anxiety that an elective c-section began to seem like a good idea. It was Giovanna who told me all about hypnobirthing and as I had used similar relaxation techniques during our fertility treatment it was something I wanted to investigate further with Hollie. I very quickly realised how much it was helping me. There is such a practical side to hypnobirthing that I wasn't expecting, and it surprised me. Hypnobirthing explains what is happening in your body as you labour and deliver your baby. I listened to meditations and visualisations every night, which helped to calm down my busy mind, and I understood that I needed to put in the work to really get the most out of it. The other part of hypnobirthing that I loved was that it included Harry. One of the best tips for Harry was to pack my hospital bag, which made total sense as he needed to know where everything was! He helped me with the breathing and relaxation techniques and also fuelled me with much-needed energy snacks!

I was nine days overdue when I went into labour and I can honestly say that giving birth to Lola was one of the happiest experiences of my life. I had affirmations filling the room, my favourite playlist on and my grandmother's hankie with lavender oil on it.

Hypnobirthing helped me to prepare for one of the biggest moments I would ever face, and I was so incredibly grateful to have the tools to help me through it. Also, I think it's really important to say that hypnobirthing doesn't mean no pain relief. I happily said 'yes, please' to an epidural! My point being that I think hypnobirthing has a stigma attached to it that means if you hypnobirth you will simply breathe your baby out. There are many reasons why interventions may be necessary, but being able to remain peaceful and calm by using hypnobirthing techniques changes the way you deal with those situations.

When I found out I was pregnant again, I didn't have the same nerves. I suppose partly because I had done it before but mainly because I knew hypnobirthing would help me through not just the big day but also the nine months before!

I feel so incredibly lucky to have met Hollie. Thanks to her I will always remember the day I gave birth to Lola as beautiful and peaceful.

CHAPTER 2
MAKING YOUR NEST

CHOOSING YOUR CAREGIVERS

One of the biggest decisions you'll make during your pregnancy is who is going to look after you. Unless you are outside of the UK or considered high-risk, you are probably receiving your antenatal care from a midwife at your local GP practice or hospital. This may be a different midwife each time, one of a small team or a named midwife that you see every time. A lot depends on what is available in your local area, but it is a good idea to do some research and find out what is available to you. This is so important because if you don't know your options you don't have any. I know I have said this before, but that is because it is true! Knowledge really is power. Different types of care will suit different types of women and families, so it is really beneficial to seek out the best support for the kind of birth experience *you* are trying to create.

For example, if you've had a previous traumatic birth experience, you may want to feel a little more held by the kind of bespoke and personal care that an independent midwife could offer, or if you have medical issues and know you need to have consultant-led care, you may want to think about hiring a doula who can bring a more holistic and nurturing energy to your environment. Remember that one size most certainly doesn't fit all, especially when it comes to pregnancy and birth. Speak to your birth partner about this too, so that they feel involved in the decision and understand your needs for labour. On the following pages are descriptions of some of the healthcare professionals you may encounter during your pregnancy.

I surround myself with positive
people who support me
and my choices.

MIDWIVES

In the UK, most women are looked after by NHS midwives during their pregnancy, birth and the immediate period beyond. When you first find out you're pregnant, you'll go along to your GP for a booking-in appointment and to register your pregnancy. You'll then be offered regular appointments with a midwife, or sometimes an obstetrician (see below). You can expect to have up to ten antenatal appointments with your NHS midwife if it's your first baby, and a few less if it's a subsequent baby. These will normally take place at either your GP surgery, a hospital or your home. While you may not see the same midwife at every appointment, they will be keeping a record of your notes, which you will be asked to keep and bring to every appointment. You will take these with you if you go into hospital to have your baby, so that the hospital midwives can understand your care so far.

OBSTETRICIAN

If you have had a previous complicated birth, have particular medical conditions or are considered high-risk, your care may be shared between a midwife and an obstetrician. An obstetrician is a doctor who specialises in pregnancy and birth and their level of involvement will depend on your personal circumstances.

CASE-LOADING MIDWIVES

Some parts of the UK offer something called case-loading (or community) midwifery within their NHS trusts. It is a free service where you will receive continued care from a named midwife throughout your pregnancy, during the birth and in the immediate postnatal period. This midwife (or one from a small team of midwives) will take all of your antenatal and postnatal appointments – often in the comfort of your home – and will be the midwife looking after you in labour. The main benefit of this style of care is that you will get continuity of care from someone you know, trust and with whom you can build a personal relationship.

INDEPENDENT MIDWIVES

Independent midwives (sometimes referred to as private midwives) are qualified midwives who are self-employed and work outside the NHS. They perform the same antenatal and postnatal clinical assessments that would happen with the NHS, but they are also available for you to contact outside of hours and can offer you longer or more flexible appointments than you may receive traditionally. This is care that you will have to pay for but in a similar way to the case-loading care mentioned above, you will establish a relationship with one or a small group of named midwives who will look after you and your family during your pregnancy, birth and the postnatal period.

You can hire independent midwives in different capacities: for the duration of your pregnancy, birth and the postnatal period, just for the birth and postnatal period, or for one-off postnatal (or prenatal) appointments to support with specific issues or concerns. Some independent midwives are experienced in helping women with twins, breech babies or those planning a VBAC (vaginal birth after caesarean). By choosing independent care, you are not opting out of NHS care and you remain entitled to all of the blood tests and scans that every woman receives. Your independent midwife can also refer you for consultant-led care or hospital admission if necessary. It's worth noting though that most independent midwives attend births at home. If you are planning to birth in a birth centre or hospital (or need to be transferred during labour), you will be looked after by a hospital midwife, and your independent midwife will then take on a support/birth partner role.

DOULA

A doula (from the Greek word meaning 'woman servant or caregiver') is an expert in birth (although not a medical professional) who can offer emotional and physical support to a woman and her birth partner before, during and after birth, in any setting. Doula Beccy Hands explains that having personal support from a close female friend or relative through labour is a tradition that many human cultures have shared for thousands of years. In today's busy world, not everyone has such a support network on hand, and this is where a doula can help.

Again, this is a service you pay for, and a doula's role is to 'mother the mother' rather than provide medical care, often working alongside the midwife and medical staff in harmony. They will offer comfort, reassurance and encouragement to a labouring mother based on her individual needs. Rather than replacing the role of the birth partner, they will be an extra person by your side – and on your side – who can help you in profound ways, however your birth unfolds. During your labour and birth, your doula will be a quiet, constant, calming presence to guide and support you through the birth of your child. Ideally you will feel unobserved but very well cared for, creating the optimum conditions for a healthy labour.

If you are considering hiring a doula, you will need to decide whether you want a birth doula (who supports you antenatally and during labour), a postnatal doula (who nurtures you in the days and weeks after you've given birth) or a doula who can combine both roles. You would also want to meet a few doulas or chat on the phone with them to find the perfect fit for your family, as this is a person who will be sharing a very intimate time with you.

WHERE TO BIRTH YOUR BABY

Just to be clear, and to reiterate what I said at the beginning of this book, there really is no right or wrong place to have your baby. Whether you choose to birth in a hospital, a birth centre or at home, what I'm talking about here is making your birthing space as private and safe as possible and setting up an environment that appeals to your primal needs as a birthing woman. Essentially, it's about making your nest.

It makes sense to start by looking at the various options you have in terms of where to have your baby. Most first-time parents in the UK choose to have their baby in a hospital, but I really want to urge you to start making decisions based on what's best for you and your baby, rather than simply doing what other people do or what you think is 'normal'. Making personal, informed decisions will contribute to your experience being positive and empowering so don't feel pressured into doing one thing over another. If being surrounded by the best of your local area's medical profession is what will make you feel most reassured and relaxed, then go for it! Don't decide on a home birth because you feel it's what you *should* be doing. Equally, if nothing sounds more comforting than giving birth surrounded by all your familiar things, then definitely explore the possibility of birthing at home. Whatever you decide, make sure you are fully informed about each option before you make your mind up. The only thing to be mindful of in terms of timing, is that you will need to let your healthcare provider know you want a home birth by week 34 in most trusts, so that they can help you get set up for this.

Essentially, it's worth considering how you think you would personally feel in each of these birth environments. Remember that when you feel most relaxed, you function in your parasympathetic nervous system (see page 59), which means your reproductive systems get the fuel they need to work comfortably and efficiently, while your baby gets a good supply of blood and oxygen. This is only compromised when your sympathetic nervous system kicks into action because you are scared or not secure in your surroundings, meaning you produce adrenaline, which is more likely to lead to intervention during labour.

Ultimately, the *best* place for you to have the *best* birth, is where *you* feel the safest and most relaxed.

To begin with though, I ask you to *unmake* your decision (if you've made one) about where you're going to have your baby. The reason for this isn't to try and change your mind, but rather to give you all the information on all the options, and then give you time to choose what feels right for you and your family. While information and advice will vary from trust to trust around the UK, over the next few pages I'm going to try to help you make sense of the current information from the NHS on choosing your birth environment.

HOSPITAL BIRTH

Most women in the UK will choose to give birth in an NHS hospital maternity unit. You'll often hear this referred to as a 'labour ward', which I think sounds off-putting. Contrary to how it sounds, you will not be on a ward of labouring women once you are in established labour. You will in fact have your own private room within the maternity unit and your care will be led by midwives unless you are high-risk or opting for consultant-led care. If there is more than one hospital in your area, you can choose which one to go to and your midwife can help you decide which hospital feels right for you.

Advantages to having your baby in hospital include having direct access to obstetricians and neonatologists should any special circumstances arise during labour or once your baby is born, having access to all pain relief options, and, for many women, feeling safer in a medical establishment. Because you'll be in your own room for established labour and the birth of your baby, you still have a good amount of control over how your environment feels and how you adapt it to feel more nest-like (which we'll talk about in more detail on page 102).

Things that may seem less appealing for some women are being in an unfamiliar, overtly medical or busy environment, the possibility of being moved to a postnatal ward once your baby is born, being looked after by midwives that you don't know, facing the pressure of hospital time frames and protocols (with regard to speed of progress in labour and specific foetal monitoring, for example), and potentially not having access to a pool if that is important to you.

MIDWIFE-LED UNITS OR BIRTH CENTRES

Midwife-led units are either completely separate from a hospital or are linked to a general hospital. Advantages include being in a less medical environment, which may not feel as intimidating, generally being in more relaxed surroundings and being looked after by a smaller team of midwives or even a midwife you have got to know during your pregnancy. Statistically there is also a lower chance of medical intervention than for women giving birth in hospital.

Things that may seem less appealing about this option for some women are the possibility of needing to transfer to a hospital should any special circumstances arise, not having direct access to pain relief (other than gas and air) and delays in accessing obstetric care should the need arise.

HOME BIRTH

If you have a straightforward pregnancy and are considered low-risk, you may like to consider having your baby at home. If you give birth at home, you'll be supported by a midwife who will be with you while you're in labour and then an additional midwife when you are ready to birth your baby. If any special circumstances arise during a home birth, your midwife will make arrangements for you to be transferred to the nearest hospital.

Home birth is a popular choice for couples who have done a hypnobirthing course because they can link the desired hormonal responses for labour with ones they naturally produce in their own home. There are additional advantages to having your baby at home, including not having to interrupt your labour to travel to hospital or a birth centre; not necessarily having to arrange childcare for other children, if you'd like them there; an increased likelihood of being looked after by a midwife who you have established a relationship with during your pregnancy; and, of course, getting into your own bed afterwards!

Things that may seem less appealing about this option for some women are the possibility of needing to transfer to a hospital if special circumstances arise and not having access to pain relief (although gas and air is available at home). Despite 'the mess' being a common worry of a home birth, your midwife can reassure you that this really isn't an issue because of the special absorbent coverings they will bring with them.

If you do decide to plan a home birth, the only things you really need at home are some old towels and a birth pool if you know you'd like to use one in labour. These can be bought online, or even second-hand if you just want to buy a new liner.

Statistically speaking, for women having their first baby, home birth slightly increases the risk of a poor outcome for the baby (from five in 1,000 for a hospital birth to nine in 1,000 – almost one per cent – for a home birth). For women having a subsequent baby, a planned home birth is as safe as having your baby in hospital or a midwife-led unit. If you do decide to plan a home birth, you can still choose to go to hospital whenever you like, so it's certainly worth thinking about if you're not sure what you'll want until the day comes!

I make informed decisions
that feel right for me
and my baby.

DECIDING WHERE TO GIVE BIRTH

When it comes to reaching a decision about where you'd like to have your baby, I would advise writing down all three options and then making a pros and cons list under each. That way you have something tangible to work with and reasons that are personal to you (rather than to other people). Sit with your lists for a few days, keep the conversation going with your birth partner, and you'll soon start to realise which option feels like the right one for you.

If you're worried about what other people will think about your choice, I have a very simple piece of advice for you: don't tell them. It is no one else's business where you decide to have your baby and remember that other people's opinions probably aren't based on quite as much knowledge and information as yours now are.

Here are some questions that you might also want to consider when thinking about where to have your baby. Discuss them with your birth partner or potential caregivers where relevant.

- What care options and places of birth are available in my area?

- Does my local hospital have a midwife-led unit, or is it only a labour ward?

- Will water or a pool be available to me?

- Will my birth partner be able to stay with me overnight after our baby is born?

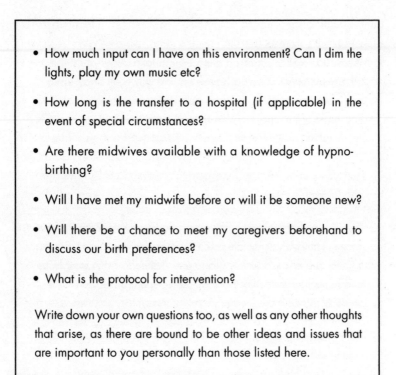

- How much input can I have on this environment? Can I dim the lights, play my own music etc?

- How long is the transfer to a hospital (if applicable) in the event of special circumstances?

- Are there midwives available with a knowledge of hypno-birthing?

- Will I have met my midwife before or will it be someone new?

- Will there be a chance to meet my caregivers beforehand to discuss our birth preferences?

- What is the protocol for intervention?

Write down your own questions too, as well as any other thoughts that arise, as there are bound to be other ideas and issues that are important to you personally than those listed here.

MAKING YOUR NEST

Wherever you decide to have your baby, there are lots of ways to make it feel calm, comfortable and familiar. Get into the habit of using some of these ideas now, during your pregnancy, to help you relax and prepare your mind for birth. That way, when the time comes, you will be able to associate the details of your environment with feeling safe and secure.

Think about appealing to all your senses for a fully immersive experience. It's a good idea to check out the space in which you will give birth too – ask your midwife if you can take a tour of the hospital or birthing centre if you are planning on having your baby there.

Helping make your 'nest' is also a really great way to get your birth partner involved so they will know what you need during labour.

LIGHTING

Interestingly, most women (and mammals) go into labour at night. This is because melatonin (a hormone your body releases at night) synergises with oxytocin to enhance the efficiency of surges. Darkness or dimly lit spaces are ideal for labour, so take this into consideration when making your nest. If you're at home, you'll be able to draw the curtains and light candles, but a similar atmosphere is also achievable in hospital or birth centre. Consider taking a portable black-out blind with you and some LED tealights/candles to create that cosy effect.

SMELLS

Essential oils are a brilliant way to calm the senses and bring about a sense of safety and relaxation during labour. If you are planning a home birth, you can use these in a diffuser or oil burner. Otherwise, splash a few drops on to a handkerchief or damp flannel. Lavender is a wonderfully calming scent, and you can start incorporating this into your bedtime routine so that it brings about similar feelings when you use it in labour. If you're travelling to hospital, having some lavender to inhale on a tissue can be a great way to keep you in your metaphorical space. (See page 183 for more on essential oils.)

COMFORT

Comfort is key in labour, as the happier and more at ease you feel physically, the more relaxed you will feel emotionally. Bear in mind that your body temperature may fluctuate during labour, so think about things that will warm you up and cool you down when necessary. A hot water bottle, microwavable heat packs, cooling eye patches or frozen flannels are a good place to start, along with a hand-held fan that your birth partner can hold. Your own pillow is also a must!

SOUNDS

Start compiling a birth playlist with your partner and make it nice and long with a good selection of music you find relaxing, loving and uplifting. Bear in mind this doesn't have to be whale sounds or an Enya soundtrack! You want music that is going to make you feel happy and at ease, so if you have a playlist from your wedding or a special event, that's a great way to generate those happy hormones on your baby's birth day. If you're having your baby in hospital, this is also a great way to zone out the noise of other people – don't forget to pop some portable speakers and headphones in your birth bag!

FEEL-GOOD SNACKS

Have a think about what food you'd like to take with you and the emotional responses these foods trigger in you. Where possible I'd avoid energy drinks that contain caffeine and focus on things that release energy more slowly. Get in a few bars of your favourite, good-quality chocolate and some luxury dried fruit and nuts. Think about your favourite smoothies and drinks too – you want to feel indulged during labour, not like you're skimping on fuel!

HYPNOBIRTHING YOUR WAY:

EXERCISE 5

Carve out some time this week to sit down with your birth partner and talk about the kind of birth environment you'd like to create, wherever you decide to have your baby. Here are some practical ideas to get the conversation going:

Creating a birth playlist
Rather than sitting in front of the television one evening, listen to music and start compiling your birth playlist.

Ask yourselves:
• What are mum's favourite songs?
• What are dad's favourite songs?
• What songs make you feel relaxed?
• What songs make you feel energised?
• What is the one song that always puts a smile on your face?

Instant relaxation
Think of things that make you feel relaxed without much effort and think about how you could draw on these in labour.

For example:

• Is there a smell that you associate with being relaxed? Could you find an essential oil or candle to replicate this? If so, start using it when you practise your face relaxation script or soft stroking massage (see pages 63 and 82), so that you begin to associate it even more deeply with relaxation.

• What's the most relaxing place you've ever visited? Find a picture of it online or a photograph you've taken and keep it visible at home. Take this with you when you go into labour and allow it to anchor you in relaxation. Try taking yourself to this place in moments of stress, too. The more you get used to using this technique to short-circuit adrenaline production now, the more effective it will be when you use it in labour.

• How and where do you respond to physical touch? I remember finding the feeling of my husband's hand on my shoulder or the side of my face completely comforting. When you feel nurtured by your birth partner, you'll produce those happy hormones that make birth work and feel more comfortable and at ease.

My baby's birth will be easy because I am so relaxed.

RELEASING FEAR

The more we understand about how the hormones we produce dictate what happens in our bodies and how we feel, the easier it is to conclude that fear is simply not good for a pregnant woman or a birthing mother.

Although it would be great if any fear surrounding pregnancy and birth just didn't exist in the first place, unfortunately – and mainly through a lifetime of social conditioning – it is likely that all pregnant women will feel a little bit fearful at some point, if only through a fear of the unknown. Please feel reassured that it is very, very normal to feel anxious about birth especially if it is something you've not done before. So don't feel like a lost cause if you've got this far and are still feeling scared.

It's what we choose to do with this fear that counts. We have three options:

1. We can either bury our heads in the sand and pretend it isn't happening, although pretending we're not scared doesn't mean the fear isn't there. When we ignore fear, it will just linger in the background and come up to bite us when labour begins, so that's not a good idea.

2. We can succumb to the fear and accept that birth is likely to be pretty horrible and anything better than that is a bonus. For this one I'd say raise your bar, ladies! You're already learning how strong and capable the system you have in place is, and to underestimate that is doing yourself a massive disservice.

3. The third option (and the one I'm suggesting we go for here) is to acknowledge what our fears are and give them the time and space they need to be heard. When we identify what we are feeling fearful of, we can work towards dealing with it, releasing the fears we don't need, and letting the ones that are okay just sit there without disturbing us too much.

Don't be afraid of your fears. Feeling scared means that you're doing something really courageous, and you are going to feel so in awe of yourself when you're holding your baby in your arms, believe me. Over the coming pages, I will show you how you can start to address any fears you may have to lead you to a place of empowerment.

I choose to birth without fear.

FEAR AND THE MIND

When addressing our fears surrounding birth, it's worth starting off by looking at the bigger picture of birth. Do you think women in less developed parts of the world have the same fears around birth?

I remember seeing footage of a group of women birthing in the Congo. There were three or four women standing together in the water, swaying and dancing and holding hands, stroking and leaning on each other. These women were in the throes of labour, and as their babies were born (with them still standing upright), they reached down to receive them and then brought them up to their chest for skin-to-skin contact. They appeared completely together and at one with what their bodies were doing, and it has always stuck with me that the narrator then said, 'These women do not experience pain because they do not *expect* to experience pain'.

In parts of the world where medicalised childbirth isn't the norm, children grow up seeing birth as a normal part of life and something that women are in control of. Pregnant women will be looked after by other women who they often know and trust, and when they labour it will normally be in familiar surroundings supported by people with whom they already have a relationship. From a young age, these are the kinds of ideas that penetrate girls' subconscious minds, meaning they expect it to be this way and respond accordingly in their own labour, i.e. they do not trigger the stressor responses that we do.

Of course, we also know that mother and infant mortality rates are higher in parts of the world where medical assistance isn't readily available. We are incredibly lucky to have the support of modern medicine when it is needed. However, it is definitely worth considering the effect of how our expectations of birth manifest into the reality of our experience.

In a similar way, have you ever experienced an animal giving birth? I remember my cat having kittens many years ago. We set up a cardboard box with some newspaper and blankets inside and popped it behind a chest of drawers. One evening, when it got dark and the house was quiet, we noticed that she was pacing around a bit, obviously looking for a safe place to labour. We stroked her gently and guided her up to the box and then left the room. We heard a bit of shuffling around and some primal cat noises and within the hour we went in to find her cleaning up four little kittens. It was so incredibly efficient and natural for her to just get on with it when she felt safe and unobserved, and women need to feel those things when they labour too.

I'm obviously not suggesting you get into a cardboard box in the spare room, but it's really worth thinking about how to make your surroundings as quiet, intimate and nest-like as possible, wherever you're going to birth your baby. Safety is key too. When we feel safe, we function in our parasympathetic state (where we produce plenty of endorphins and oxytocin, see page 149 for more on this), so start thinking about things that make you feel this way. Refer back to pages 102 on making your nest and creating an optimal birth environment. But also remember that feeling relaxed as you approach birth also lies within your internal control.

TAKING CONTROL

Most women tend to be in a sympathetic state when they go into labour. They are, therefore, producing adrenaline, and this is the hormone that inhibits birth working comfortably and efficiently (see page 149). So why *are* we producing adrenaline when we go into labour? Where does the fear come from?

To start with, I want you to take a moment to think about your own feelings surrounding childbirth. Consider where any fears you may have come from, and who or what has influenced them. Jot them down on a piece of paper before reading on.

As a starting point, I'm sure you'll agree that our media has a lot to answer for in terms of the way it portrays birth. Think about what birth looks like on TV and in films. The characteristics are likely to include a highly medicalised environment, bright lights, a mum who is on her back screaming and sweating, a useless or irritating birth partner, a stressful/panicked atmosphere, lots of staff or authority figures in white coats and, of course, other people being in control while mum is passive and doing as she's told.

Consider that description for a moment. It doesn't do particularly well in portraying an event which is in fact natural, empowering, safe and physically efficient, does it?

In some antenatal classes or groups there is also a reinforcement of the pain concept with a lot of focus on pain relief and 'getting through' the experience of birth. You are therefore prepped to go into an experience assuming you're going to be in pain before you even know what the sensations of labour feel like. I'm by no means denouncing birth education programmes, and I know that some women genuinely do want to birth their baby with the aid of pain relief, but should we be endorcing the general assumption that it is going to be necessary?

Another factor that may increase our fear of birth is the idea of not being in control. In our day-to-day lives we are used to having control over so much of what we experience, but giving birth is still a big unknown. Even if you have already had a baby before, each birth is different. So it is very common for women to adopt a 'worst-case scenario' approach to birth. Unsurprisingly, this is not helpful in creating a positive experience and mindset as you prepare for birth.

HYPNOBIRTHING YOUR WAY:

EXERCISE 6

With all this in mind, I'm going to set you a very important piece of homework. I want you and your birth partner to both make a list of all of your fears around birth. Bear in mind it doesn't just have to be about the birth itself, but it can also include any anxiety that comes to mind when you think about becoming parents.

You can each make a list as long as you like, then sit together and take turns to go through each item on your list, discussing each one openly and honestly. When you've both finished, I want you to cross anything off your list that feels smaller than when you started. Then I want you to shred or burn your pieces of paper to represent letting go of fears that no longer serve you or the wonderful, safe experience that lies ahead of you. This will help you to start reprogramming your subconscious minds to accept birth as the normal, efficient, safe event that it is.

It's important to remember that as you go through your pregnancy, your fears may change (and so might your partner's), so repeat this exercise whenever you're feeling twinges of anxiety or fear about what's ahead. Burying your fears can distract the conscious mind for a while, but they will still be sitting there in your subconscious if you don't take responsibility for addressing them. I genuinely think this is one of the most valuable exercises you can do as you prepare for the birth of your child. Not only will it bring you closer as a couple – sharing your vulnerabilities and supporting each other is a wonderfully intimate thing – but it will also mean that your subconscious won't trigger that automatic adrenaline response when you go into labour, because it will have relearned that birth is safe.

DEXTER'S BIRTH
SHARED BY RACHEL ELLIS-BARBER

Childbirth. Even the word to me conjured up thoughts of surgical procedures and hospital environments where women are screaming and men are wringing their hands in despair.

I had heard my three older sisters regale, with gruesome detail, a blow-by-blow account of their experiences and it filled me with dread. Why is it that people love to tell a 'bad' birth experience but you never get to hear the positive ones? It must mean that there is no such thing as a good childbirth then, surely?

Once my husband and I had navigated the ups and downs of 'trying for a baby' we found ourselves finally pregnant. This is the exact point that the self-doubt crept in. It's going to be awful, I told myself. At that same time and by a stroke of good luck a very good friend had started a course in hypnobirthing and was giving me the low-down on what it was all about. It sounded a bit airy-fairy until she explained that in actual fact it is all very logical. I googled a bit, chatted to my husband who was surprisingly onboard from the get-go and off we went to our first class.

We learned more about the reality of childbirth in that first class than I had heard from a lifetime of birth stories. We finished the course, practised as much as we could and felt armed with everything we could possibly need for a good birth. The reality was even better than I could have imagined. It was hard – the hardest thing I have ever done – but at no point did I ever doubt that my body and my baby couldn't do it. My husband played a huge part in the whole thing. He kept me calm when I was starting to wobble, he just had everything in control. We planned a home birth and he was checking in with the midwife regularly. We were quickly building the birth pool between contractions (there's nothing like a bit of flat pack building to take your mind off labour). When we both decided she needed to come, I was already 8cm dilated and Max was born shortly after. It was an experience like no other. I was tucked up in my bed with my baby, a cup of tea and crumpets within minutes, while the midwives and my husband were acting out a comedy sketch in the living room as one the midwives nearly slipped in the pool and the emptying hose dislodged and flooded our flat!

After Max's birth I had the usual questions: 'which hospital were you in?' and 'was it just awful?'. My response every time was 'oh, no it was pretty mindblowing and really amazing – I had him at home'. The reactions varied but a lot of people would say 'you're brave!' That filtered into my conscience and when I became pregnant again I started to doubt everything. Was I really just lucky? I couldn't possibly have a good experience a second time.

We did a hypnobirthing refresher course with Hollie and practised as much as we could with a toddler in tow. I had a second, lovely but very different home birth. Kelly, my midwife, visited me throughout my pregnancy and was there for the birth. The surges were consistent and getting stronger throughout the day. It was also my husband's birthday so all our lovely plans for a leisurely lunch and cinema date flew out of the window!

We had dispatched our toddler to Grandma to avoid the inevitable 'can I get in the pool mummy, where are my goggles?'. Kelly came to check on how things were progressing but thinking I was in for a long labour I asked her to come back when things were really happening. We had yet another birth pool faux pas when my husband realised he'd got the wrong nozzle for the hose and hot-footed it to the local DIY shop in a blind panic. I was 10cm when she arrived the second time and she ushered me into the pool. The water didn't help me as much as it did the first time as I had left it a bit too late. It was a much more intense and very quick birth in the end and completely different to my first experience, but I felt calm throughout and never doubted that my body could do it.

I firmly believe there was nothing lucky about my experience. I kept all my options open and was fully prepared to go to hospital if I needed to, but the reality was that we got out what we put in with our practice, and with an amazing birth team of my husband and the exceptional community midwives I was able to have the births I wanted.

WRITING YOUR BIRTH PREFERENCES

From the moment you find out you're pregnant, you have a whole host of decisions to make about the journey ahead. Being well informed means that you are able to make the best decisions for you and your baby at each stage of your pregnancy and birth – and beyond!

Of course, we would all like to think that pregnancy and birth unfolds without any complications, and while for most women this is true, it's really important that we equip ourselves to navigate different turns that the journey might take in a calm and confident way.

One of the best ways to be clear in what you want is to get things down on paper by writing down some birth preferences. You will probably be familiar with the term 'birth plan' but I prefer to keep away from the word 'plan' as it always feels limiting and final. Thinking of these ideas as preferences instead keeps the door open for change.

There are lots of things to consider when writing up your preferences – and I have provided some good starting points on the next page. But I want to highlight two items, which will require a bit more research on your part. These are the vitamin K injection that is offered to newborns, and whether you choose to have a natural or managed delivery of the placenta. Speak to your midwife about these two things and make sure you understand the benefits and risks of all options so that you have the complete information you need to make an informed decision. It's also worth knowing that if, for example, your baby needs to be born by caesarean section, there are still plenty of items on your birth preferences that you can remain in control of.

I recommend printing off a few copies of your birth preferences. That way they remain an active part of your labour, and your birth partner can advocate them on your behalf by communicating with your midwives and keeping the conversation and rapport open and supportive. Essentially, whenever you need to make an informed decision about your care, there's a really simple acronym to remember that will help. The acronym is BRAIN!

Benefits – what are the benefits of this option for me and my baby?

Risks – what are the risks of this option for me and my baby?

Alternatives – what are my other options?

Instinct – what does my gut say?

Nothing – what happens if I choose to do nothing? (Be time-specific with this one, i.e. choosing to do nothing for one hour or one day, depending on the relevance to the suggested intervention.)

If you have the answers to all of those questions, you will be able to make a decision that feels right for you and your baby. That is what's going to line you up for a truly positive and empowering experience, regardless of how your baby chooses to enter the world.

A TEMPLATE FOR WRITING YOUR BIRTH PREFERENCES

1. Include your basic information at the top of your birth preferences so that your details, and those of your birth partner, can be easily located.
Mother's name:

Mother's phone number:

Birth partner's name:

Birth partner's phone number:

Intended birth place:

2. Write a short paragraph about where you intend to give birth and the type of environment you are trying to create, for example:

We would like to create a calm, quiet environment for our birth. This includes, where possible: dimmed lighting, our own music, essential oils, quiet voices and no unnecessary people in the room. We are/aren't happy to have students present.

3. Write a brief outline of how you intend to use hypnobirthing. Also, include a word about how you'd like your caregivers' support on this.

We are using hypnobirthing techniques and would like a natural birth with as little intervention as possible. In the absence of a medical emergency, we would choose patience over intervention or any procedure that could unnecessarily stand in the way of having the most natural birth possible. We will use the word surge instead of contraction, and pressure instead of pain, and would appreciate your support with this. We would like an active labour, with the freedom to walk and move around, as well as to eat and drink.

4. Include how you feel about having vaginal examinations to monitor your progress throughout labour. Choose one of the below:

I am happy to have regular vaginal examinations.

I would only like vaginal examinations if there's a cause for concern/medical reason.

I do not want any vaginal examinations.

5. What kind of monitoring would you like for the baby's heartbeat? Choose from the below:
I would like continual sonar foetal monitoring.

I would like regular but not continual foetal monitoring using a hand-held Doppler/stethoscope.

6. Consider how you would like to move around during labour and birth. Where possible, I would like to be upright and forward-leaning rather than lying on my back. I would like to use:
Squatting
Leaning forward/over bed etc.
A birth pool
A birth stool
Standing, supported by my partner

7. Add any thoughts about whether or not you'd like to use water during labour. Consider these options:
I do not intend to use water during my birth.

I would like to use the birth pool throughout labour.

I would like to use baths/showers during the earlier stages of labour and the pool at the end of labour and for birth.

If possible, I would like to give birth in the water.

8. Outline how you'd like to approach pain relief during labour.

I am happy to be offered pain relief.

I do not want to be offered pain relief.

If I ask for pain relief, I am open to using:

- Gas and air
- Pethidine
- Epidural
- Spinal block

If I ask for pain relief, I do not want to use:

- Gas and air
- Pethidine
- Epidural
- Spinal block

9. Consider how you'd like to be supported in birthing your baby.

I would like to birth my baby using mother-led breathing rather than midwife-directed pushing. I want to follow the lead of my body and I do not want to rush the process in the absence of a medical issue. I am/am not happy for trainee doctors/students to observe the birth.

10. Outline what you'd like to happen immediately after birth. Consider the below:

I would like me/my partner to receive our baby.

I would like my partner to announce the sex.

I would like to wait until the umbilical cord has stopped pulsating before cutting it.

My partner would like to cut our baby's cord if possible.

I would like immediate skin-to-skin contact with my baby.

I would like the vernix to be absorbed into baby's skin (no cleaning or rubbing).

I would like support in establishing breastfeeding.

I would like our environment kept as calm as possible.

I would like my baby to be given vitamin K by injection.

I would like my baby to be given vitamin K orally.

I do not want my baby to be given vitamin K at all if they have been born without intervention.

11. How would you like to birth your placenta?
I would like a natural third stage in the absence of an emergency.

I would like a managed third stage.

I would like to keep my placenta.

12. Outline what you'd like to do in the event of special circumstances.
I would like any suggested intervention to be fully explained to me and my partner. Unless an emergency arises, we are happy to be patient with labour rather than rush it. In the event of an assisted delivery, we would like as many of our preferences considered as possible.

13. If you are planning a caesarean section or know there is a chance you may need one if labour takes an unexpected turn, it is a good idea to write some preferences to make sure it is still a really positive birth experience. Consider the below:

- As I will be relaxed and within my birthing body, in the first instance any questions should be addressed to my birth partner.
- I would like my partner/birth partner to be present throughout.
- Where possible we would like to create a calm environment, with our own relaxation music playing, either through a player or headphones.
- We realise the need for bright lights during the operation but we ask for lights to be dimmed when baby is passed to me.
- I'd like the drip to be in my non-dominant arm so I can hold my baby as soon as possible without interference.
- Where possible, I'd like delivery of the baby to be slowed to allow the fluid to be squeezed out of baby's lungs.
- I'd like to have skin-to-skin contact with my baby straight after birth so please position ECG dots away from the front of my chest. Where possible I'd like undisturbed skin-to-skin for at least an hour after birth to allow optimum oxytocin release.
- I'd like delayed cord clamping where possible.
- I'd like all midwifery jobs to be done without separating me from my baby.

14. Make sure to include anything else you'd like to communicate.

STAYING POSITIVE

Remember that your birth preferences document is a chance to communicate your preferences rather than to set in stone a plan that doesn't offer flexibility. The first thing on your birth preferences should be an open mind. A positive birth experience means you feeling in control and calm. This can be maintained however your labour unfolds if you think ahead and work as a team with your birth partner who will be protecting your space and advocating for you along the way.

My advice would be to start jotting down some ideas for your birth preferences early on, so that they have time and space to evolve as your pregnancy progresses and you refine your idea of what a positive experience looks like to *you*. Ask your midwife any questions you have about how things work in different birth environments, so you get a clearer idea on how you can all work together so that you feel supported in the best possible way.

On a practical note, keep your birth preferences to short sentence/bullet point form and make it no more than one A4 sheet of paper. Make it easy for your caregivers to read, and take at least three copies with you, in the event that there may be shift changes while you are being looked after.

HYPNOBIRTHING YOUR WAY:

EXERCISE 7

Perhaps now that your mind has been busy working its way through all of these options, it would be a good opportunity to revisit your calm breathing (see page 60) to still your thoughts and quieten the mind before you relax for a few moments.

Stop whatever you're doing and, whether you're on the bus, in bed or in a coffee shop, just take a few moments to notice the rhythm of your breath, and start inhaling the word peace and exhaling the word tension.

Breathe in and out all through the nose, trying to make your exhale slightly longer than your inhale if this is comfortable for you. Notice any tension that may have crept into your face, neck or shoulders, and breathe into these places as you just release and let go. Close your eyes if you feel comfortable doing so or keep them open but relaxed and just breathe for a few minutes. Inhaling peace, and exhaling tension. All is well.

CHAPTER 3
WAITING FOR YOUR BABY

UNDERSTANDING DUE DATES

Ultimately, your baby will be born when your baby is ready, and the more relaxed you are in your approach to this, the more readily you'll be producing the very hormones that enable the beautiful process to begin. It's always been interesting to me that hypnobirthing couples are less likely to choose induction as a result of 'going overdue' because their babies arrive well inside their due time. The reason for this is quite simple: as opposed to feeling terrified about what's ahead, they feel relaxed, at ease, and ready for their babies to be born, knowing that they have the tools to enjoy their baby's birth calmly and in an empowered way. This feeling triggers the release of endorphins and oxytocin, the hormones that pave the way for labour to begin on its own. Being open and relaxed about when your baby might arrive is key.

Never has anything so vague been so heavily obsessed over than due dates, so I think it's important that I bust some myths around this elusive date and help you to approach your baby's due time in a more relaxed way.

When you find out you're pregnant, you'll go along to your GP and by giving them the first day of your last menstrual period (which many women aren't always completely sure of), they'll calculate your baby's estimated due date (EDD), which will be 40 weeks from the date you give. This date will be revised at your 12-week scan, where your baby's measurements will be taken into consideration to help gauge gestation.

Even from this simple explanation, I imagine you can see how the EDD approach is flawed. For a start, and as mentioned, many women don't accurately know the first day of their last period, meaning they take a close guess and a date is generated accordingly. The EDD is also calculated based on an average 28-day cycle, which many women don't have either. You're probably well aware that anything from 21 to 35 days is a completely normal cycle length, and that means women's bodies and hormones are varying by a whopping two weeks at the very least.

When you look at it this way, you can see how strange it is to expect all women to carry a baby for exactly 40 weeks. In fact, anything between 37–42 weeks is a completely normal time in which your baby can be born happily and healthily, and more importantly, ready. This is why in hypnobirthing we tend to refer to it as your due time instead (also see page 17).

Given that it's normally other people that obsess over your due date more than you will, a good tip is to add two weeks on to the EDD you've been given and offer that up as your 'due date' going forward. Chances are, you'll have had your baby by then and it stops the 'any news?' dialogue starting too early, which let's face it, isn't helpful to anyone.

┌　　　　　　　　　　　　　　　　　　┐

My baby will arrive when
the time is right.

└　　　　　　　　　　　　　　　　　　┘

PRACTICE SURGES

Practice surges, otherwise known as Braxton Hicks, are sporadic uterine waves or cramps that women sometimes experience in the second or third trimester of their pregnancies. They happen when the muscles of the uterus start to stretch and contract in preparation for labour. They may vary in intensity from barely noticeable to uncomfortable, and if you experience the latter, you can use your Calm and Open Breath techniques (see pages 60 and 166) to ease the sensations, exactly as you'll do in labour. During the later stages of pregnancy, these can sometimes be triggered by a full bladder which may create more discomfort, so be sure to go to the toilet regularly, even if you're only releasing very little! Essentially they are brilliant sign that your body is starting to warm up for its work during labour and are, of course, a great opportunity to practise your techniques and tune into how your muscles are working.

VISUALISATION

Visualisation is a great tool for taking yourself somewhere peaceful and safe, even if your actual surroundings don't feel that way. It can be a brilliant technique to use throughout your pregnancy and during your labour, especially in times of stress or disruption. Because it's probably not something you'll be used to having done before, it can take some practice for visualisation to become effective, but the good news is that it's something that can be practised anytime, anywhere, as of now.

When you first try visualisations, you may feel like your mind is going crazy, distracting you and asking lots of questions. That's just because it feels a bit alien right now and you're likely to be a bit suspicious of what on earth you're doing! But those feelings will subside the more you practise.

MAGGIE'S BIRTH
SHARED BY KATY BAKER

Maggie was born on 21 June 2016 during the full moon, and a healthy 8lbs 5oz, at 42 weeks plus 3 days.

I had a show in the early hours of the morning then felt a 'pop'. We were planning a home birth – we had the pool, lights, aromatherapy oils, play list, affirmations and a fridge full of snacks. I was concerned the fluid was a browny/green colour though. At that point my surges were really strong and I had been vomiting quite badly. I was starting to worry when Chris started playing my relaxation MP3. Immediately I felt calmer. As soon as I heard 'I follow my instincts and make informed decisions that are right for me and my baby' I knew what I had to do. We made our way to hospital.

The midwives identified the fluid as meconium. Maggie was showing signs of foetal distress; I took a deep breath and asked for an epidural. I could see where I was heading and needed to be as calm and pain-free as possible to mentally and physically deal with the cascade of interventions that were about to ensue. I was given a mobile epidural and concentrated on staying calm and switching off from the fact I was now at entirely the other end of the spectrum from what I had planned for our birth. Chris set up the room and put some lavender oil in our diffuser and I continued to listen to my

MP3, breathing through the surges and down to my baby to keep her calm.

Maggie's heart rate was causing concern. Outside the room there was talk of instrumental delivery or more likely a c-section. Chris was amazing and shielded me from all of this, only telling me what I needed to know in a calm and positive way.

I wasn't progressing so was given a hormone drip. By this time I was in my own world, doing my best to breathe calmness and love down to my baby. The consultant looking after me was gunning to deliver without a c-section. I visualised my baby being birthed. In the short time it took to transfer me to theatre, I had fully dilated and mustered all my strength to push. Before I knew it, Maggie was out (with a little help from a ventouse) and on my chest. I had done it!

The effect that hypnobirthing had on my birth experience was profound. The course really helped me connect with Maggie and be as informed as possible about what lay ahead. It also taught us that although plans can change mindset doesn't have to. The techniques we learned, teamed with the amazing support of my husband, meant that although my birth path changed I have nothing but positive thoughts of my whole experience and would do it all over again 100 times over. I owned my birthing experience and I am immensely proud of it.

HYPNOBIRTHING YOUR WAY:

EXERCISE 8

First of all, I want you to think – in your conscious mind – of a time and place where you felt really happy and relaxed. Maybe it's a moment from your childhood, a home comfort or somewhere you've been on holiday. Don't worry if a few spring to mind, you can practise with all of them as the weeks go by, but for now, just settle on one place. Take a few deep breaths and really try and picture what this place or moment looks like.

What I'd like you to do now is to start switching on all of your senses in this safe and happy place. What does it smell like here? Can you smell food being prepared? Can you smell the sea or the scent of other people? Flowers? Fresh grass? And what do you hear? Can you hear waves lapping against a shore? Leaves blowing in a breeze? Birds and wildlife? A familiar song? What does it feel like here? Is it warm or cool? What are you standing or sitting on? Asking yourself these questions in your mind will help transport you more fully to the feelings of comfort that this place can offer you, and which you'll revisit often.

When you start to have a clearer idea of what this safe and happy place looks and feels like for you (you could even have a go at drawing it or pulling up a photograph of it if that helps), I want you to set aside five minutes every day to take yourself there.

At first, do it in the same place every day – when you wake up in the morning or get into bed in the evening can be a good place. Start with some calm breathing, close your eyes, and drift off to this wonderful place in your mind. As this becomes easier, try having a go when you're in different places – on the Tube, in the office, in the park or other public space. Nobody will know what you're doing, so don't feel shy. Just find a place to sit down, close your eyes and breathe. Before you know it, you'll be able to drift off to this tranquil place at a moment's notice, and it will then be second nature for you to use in labour.

Visualisation can be a particularly good tool to use alongside other hypnobirthing techniques should your labour take any unexpected turns. Let's say you need to transfer from a planned home birth to hospital, or that intervention you were hoping to avoid becomes necessary. Using the visualisation technique means you can calm your mind quickly and stop it from entering panic mode where your body produces adrenaline and works against the process of birth.

The calmer you are, the calmer your baby will be, so maintaining this sense of peace, even in trickier times, will have such a positive effect on your experience. I remember when I was taken down to theatre for my c-section with Oscar, I closed my eyes, used my calm breathing and took myself off to the mountains while everyone was getting things ready around me. Because we'd been in a still and quiet environment up until that point the flapping around was making me anxious, so visualising a quiet place meant I could escape the business of what was happening around me and remain relaxed and ready to meet my baby.

REST, NEST AND NURTURE

The last weeks of pregnancy can seem like an eternity when you're waiting to meet your baby, but as we all know, a watched pot never boils. Remember that anything between 37–42 weeks is a completely normal time to have your baby, so even when you reach your full-term mark at 37 weeks, you could still have over a month to wait before you're holding your baby.

Obsessing over these days is a pointless activity, as it just creates tension in the mind and stops your thoughts from being peaceful. Rather than crossing days off the calendar impatiently, try and approach this time as a chance to really deepen your hypnobirthing practice, withdraw yourself from external pressures and enjoy the last few sacred moments of you and your baby being one. I like to think of this as the rest, nest and nurture stage – a time so magical and unique, as you prepare to transition from one life to another. Here are some ways to take your mind off waiting for your baby to make an appearance.

REST

- Now that you're on maternity leave, schedule a nap into your day. No this isn't being indulgent or lazy, it's letting your body take the time it needs to recharge. You are carrying around a human being so of course you feel heavy and tired. This is the answer! If you have a little one already, put the TV on, have a snuggle with them on the sofa and doze as they watch!

- Go to bed earlier. There is no shame in getting into bed at the same time as your child – I still do it one night a week and my son is seven! Remember that sleep before midnight is more restorative than the hours after, so get your eye mask on and catch some zzz while you can.

• On the days that naps and early nights aren't feasible, take a long, warm bath while listening to your Affirmations MP3 (see page 12). Let your body stop for a while by just lying down and listening, tuning into your breath and talking internally to your baby.

NEST

• Start thinking about life after your baby arrives. Use this time to tick things off the life admin list. This could include things like setting up a regular online shop, writing and addressing some birthday cards for the next few months so they're ready to go, getting your finances in order (such as any child benefit you may be entitled to) or downloading your favourite box sets so they're all set up for the early days.

• Wash your baby's clothes and put them away so that you haven't got to faff around with packets and packaging when they arrive.

• Batch cook some of your favourite meals to keep in the freezer. Dishes that don't take too much prep on the other side are ideal – think fish pies, stews, soups, tagines and pasta sauces. Ask friends and family to help you with this too.

NURTURE

• Set aside some time to properly pamper and nurture yourself. This could be getting a haircut, a pedicure or a massage – whatever it is that feels like a treat for you! Remember that alternative therapies such as reflexology or acupuncture (see pages 72–81) can have a very good impact on getting your body (and mind) primed and ready for birth.

• Make sure your partner is looking after you. I taught a lovely couple once and mum's partner had set up little treats for her for every day she went past her EDD. They were ideas like a cinema ticket, a manicure voucher and lunch with a friend. If mum wasn't in labour that day she had something lovely to take her mind off waiting, and if she missed it, it was because things had started. Win-win! (No pressure, partners . . .)

• Make extra time for your hypnobirthing practice. Use your breathing techniques regularly throughout the day (see pages 60 and 166) and listen to your Affirmations and Relaxation MP3s more often than you have been so far (see page 12). Practise taking yourself to your happy place that we talked about earlier (see page 133). Essentially, the more relaxed and happy you feel, the more likely it is that labour will start.

NATURAL NUDGES

As your estimated due date approaches, or maybe even passes, it is natural to start to feel a little anxious. But remember how far you have come and how much good work you have already done. There are lots of things you can be doing at home to give labour the best chance of starting naturally.

Here are some of the things we call 'natural nudges':
- Reflexology and acupuncture
  See pages 72–76 for more details on how these therapies can help get your birthing body ready for labour.

- Releasing fear
  Remember that adrenaline has the power to inhibit labour from starting. Revisit the fear release exercise on page 113. Remember that it's very normal for your fears to be different now from what they might have been a few months ago. Go back and write down your anxieties and talk about them with your birth partner. This can have a profound effect on how the subconscious mind feels about starting the process of labour. Remember it needs to feel like it's 'safe' to release your baby!

- Relaxing in a warm bath
  Put on your Affirmations MP3 (see page 12), diffuse some essential oils and enjoy a long, warm bath. Enjoy the weightlessness that the water offers you and your bump. Close your eyes and practise the visualisation techniques you learned earlier in this chapter (see page 130).

- Clary sage essential oil
  Please note that this must not be used before 37 weeks' gestation. Diffuse this with an electric diffuser, or inhale some from a handkerchief or flannel. It's quite strong, so don't douse your house in it before you realise you don't like the smell!

- Sex, intimacy and climax

  Remember that whenever we have sex, climax or share intimacy with the person we love, we produce the hormones endorphins and oxytocin. These are the exact hormones that blend to make birth work, so now is the time to connect with your birth partner in a deeper way. Hugs before drugs.

- Eat dates

  Some midwives advise women in their care to eat six dates a day from 36 weeks of pregnancy. Researchers have found that dates have an oxytocin-like effect on the body, which can help to stimulate the uterus.

- Laughter

  Yes! When we laugh we produce those happy hormones – endorphins – which inhibits the production of adrenaline, making a natural start to labour more likely. Watch some light-hearted funny TV. Feeling relaxed, safe and having a laugh are all good tonics for the anxiety that can start creeping in during the last days of pregnancy.

- Visualisation

  Now that you've learned how to visualise (see page 130), you can manifest anything you like in your mind. Try visualising holding your baby in your arms. What do they look like? What colour hair do they have? Do they look like you or your partner? Talk to your baby too – tell them it's safe and that you are ready to meet them.

- Get your birth partner involved
Ask them to give you some soft stroking massage and read the face relaxation script to you (see pages 82 and 63). Don't worry, not at the same time! This will get you super used to using these tools for when you are in labour and they can even help labour begin with all the endorphins they will help you produce!

- Dance!
Put your birth playlist on and have a dance. Dancing is great for loosening up the hips and pelvis and allowing baby's head to engage down into your pelvis. It also makes us feel good!

- Listen to your MP3s
Try to listen to your Affirmations MP3 at least twice a day and your Relaxation MP3 when you go to bed at night and when you rest during the day. Naps are where it's at!

- Recite your affirmations
Talk to your baby and say out loud that you can do this, because you really, really can!

- Pack and repack your birth bag
Double check to make sure it has everything in it you need. It's a good idea for your partner to pack your bag for you so they will be able to easily access whatever you need during labour.

- Get out in nature
Going for a walk every day can help put you in touch with how capable we are and connected we are with the world around us.

Bear in mind of course that these natural nudges aren't going to start labour unless your mind, body and baby are ready. Remember, your baby knows how and when to be born. Labour will happen when the time is right, so trust the process and relax.

I am one day closer to
holding my baby in
my arms.

PART TWO

THE BIRTH

When we start to switch our mindset and realise that birth begins from the moment we become pregnant, we are able to slowly remove the anxiety around the build-up to this one big day. Preparing our mind and body over a much longer period, gives us a better chance for a positive and empowering experience of birth. With every day that passes, you get closer to meeting your baby and you can use this time to equip yourself with an incredible set of tools and wisdom.

Try to think of the process of labour and birth as a manifestation of all of the hard work that has come before: the time you have taken to conceive your baby, the weeks and months of growing him or her and those final days of waiting and anticipation of what lies ahead.

It is one of life's most beautiful and sacred journeys. The more fully you immerse yourself in each moment, the more connected to your body and baby you will become and the more you will trust your maternal instinct as your life as a mother unfolds.

Moving towards your baby's birth day with a supportive and informed birth partner will make your journey all the more rewarding. Feeling safe and protected will mean you are able to surrender to the physical and emotional demands of becoming a mother. Your birth partner is really *not* a bystander, but rather the enabler and advocator of these profound emotional depths. Connecting during your pregnancy and working through labour and birth as the incredible team you have become will unite you in a very powerful way. I promise you that the time and effort you put into this will pay off, so talk about your experiences regularly – and by that, I mean your hopes, fears and everything in between. Practise together on a daily basis, lean on each other and respect and value each other's contribution to the birth of your baby.

Finally, I want you to remember that birthing your baby does not mean your baby has to come out of your vagina. Birthing your baby means bringing them into the world, however that may be. Be open to the way in which your baby chooses to enter this life and know that it is your calmness and confidence that will make your baby feel safe and you feel empowered. There is no such thing as a *perfect* birth, so let your focus be on creating a positive one. It is yours for the taking.

CHAPTER 4
UNDERSTANDING
THE PROCESS

GETTING YOUR MIND READY FOR BIRTH

Hopefully by now you're starting to realise that birth is as much a psychological experience as a physical one. Yes, your muscles are doing the hard graft, but it's your emotional state, and the hormones you produce as a consequence, that will dictate whether these muscles work with ease or tension.

The role of hypnobirthing is in teaching us how to be in better control of the way our body responds when labour begins. We know that when we are scared or stressed we produce adrenaline which triggers the fight, flight or freeze response. Blood and oxygen are diverted to our defence systems and *away* from our uterus. Without the fuel it needs, the uterus tenses, creating pain and distressing mother and baby. This all feeds back in to our initial societal fears that birth is painful, and we then carry on producing adrenaline to 'protect' us.

This process is a very simple cycle of fear, tension and pain, and one that I'm here to help you understand and avoid.

Fear
We fear that birth will be painful so our body produces adrenaline to 'protect' us.

Tension
Adrenaline triggers a fight, flight or freeze response, directing blood and oxygen away from the uterus, which causes the muscles to tense.

Pain
Tense muscles in the uterus causes pain, which 'confirms' our fear that birth is painful.

We do not need to produce adrenaline when we birth our baby. It is not a helpful hormone to have in the birth room and all of our efforts should be focused on keeping it at bay. The simplest way to do this is to turn your attention towards producing endorphins. We cannot produce adrenaline alongside endorphins, so think of endorphins as your secret weapon and your super power. Let's have a closer look at the role of these hormones in birth and the role they play.

THE HORMONES OF BIRTH
There are three hormones that we need to understand when it comes to birth. They are adrenaline, endorphins and oxytocin. We can produce endorphins and oxytocin at the same time, but never alongside adrenaline. This point is key in understanding how to control our hormones during labour and birth.

CYCLE OF
FEAR, TENSION, PAIN

FEAR

We fear that birth will be painful so our body produces adrenaline to 'protect' us

Adrenaline triggers a fight, flight or freeze response, directing blood and oxygen away from the uterus, which causes the muscles to tense.

Tense muscles in the uterus cause pain, which 'confirms' our fear that birth is painful.

PAIN

TENSION

Adrenaline is the hormone we release in conditions of stress. Its primary role is to keep us safe and prepare our body for the fight, flight or freeze response. We are capable of producing adrenaline very quickly and when that happens, blood and oxygen are directed to our defence systems. This means an increased heart rate and blood pressure, expanding passages in the lungs, dilating the pupils, maximising blood glucose levels for the brain and diverting blood flow to our arms and legs (so that we become stronger and faster). Common physical symptoms of adrenaline are an acceleration of heart and lung action, feeling hot and cold, shaking, stomach pain and sweating, among others. When we produce adrenaline, we feel on high alert and ready for action.

Endorphins are the happy hormones and we release these to help us relax and alleviate stress. Endorphins are our body's natural pain relief and act in a similar way to morphine (endorphins are actually stronger than morphine). We produce endorphins when we feel relaxed and happy, when we sleep or deeply rest, when we laugh and exercise and when we experience pleasure. We can also produce endorphins when we eat dark chocolate or certain other foods, and when we use calming aromatherapy oils such as lavender. Common physical symptoms of endorphins are feeling physically relaxed and emotionally secure, feeling safe, at ease and happy. Think of endorphins as your natural high!

Oxytocin is the hormone we produce when we feel safe and loved. It is the hormone of intimacy and trust. We all produce oxytocin when we orgasm and women also produce it to birth their babies and breastfeed them. It helps us to create strong bonds with one another and improves our ability to interact socially. We produce oxytocin when we are intimate with other people – when we kiss, cuddle, have eye contact, hold hands, have sex, use physical touch and so on. We produce it when we feel safe, loved and unobserved.

HORMONES IN EVERYDAY LIFE

Let's have a think about when we might produce these hormones in our everyday lives. Visualising how each one feels will make it easier for you to train your body to activate each one when you need to. Remember that you are already completely capable of producing these hormones and do so very regularly. Now it's time to become more conscious about how you use them and to learn how to manage them, so that you are in better control of how your body responds when you go into labour.

Adrenaline	Endorphins	Oxytocin
Public speaking	Exercise	Intimacy
Watching horror films	Eating dark chocolate	Cuddling
Extreme sports	Laughing	Deep breathing
Danger/threat	Sex and orgasm	Listening to music
An emotional shock	Dancing	Walking outside

The next time you experience one of the above, notice what happens in your body and how it feels. What does it feel like physically and emotionally? How does it affect your breathing? How long does the feeling last? Understanding these hormones and how it feels when your body produces them is a key component of hypnobirthing. By getting to know how they feel, you can learn to have greater control over them. Becoming more in tune with how your body reacts and your power to influence it will have a huge impact on your experience of birth.

CONTROLLING ADRENALINE

Remember that the adrenaline response is something that your body is doing, not something that is being done *to you*. This means you have the power to control it and ultimately stop your body producing adrenaline and instead boost endorphins ready for birth. The more you practise this, the easier it becomes to do. Start practising now so that by the time it comes to the birth you are able to have control over your responses. I want you to become actively aware of adrenaline responses in your body and to pick a tool to short-circuit adrenaline production and return you to a state of calm. Here are a couple of examples:

1. Imagine that you are about to cross a road. Thinking it's clear, you step out but realise that a car is coming towards you and it makes you jump. This will trigger your body's adrenaline response. Notice those feelings of breathlessness and physical tension.

Short-circuit tool: Step back on to the pavement, take a deep breath in through your nose and out through your mouth. Relax your shoulders, shake out your hands and arms, and then use a few calm breaths to re-establish a sense of calm.

2. You've had a rubbish day at work and it all just seems too much. You get home and feel impatient with your partner and don't know quite what to do with yourself or how to relax.

Short-circuit tool: Rather than reaching for your phone or switching the TV on, go and lie on your bed and put on your Relaxation MP3 (see page 12) or ask your partner to read the face relaxation script (see page 63) to you.

HYPNOBIRTHING YOUR WAY:
EXERCISE 9

In a notebook, start to write down some everyday examples of when you notice your adrenal reactions and how you manage to short-circuit them. When you look back in the weeks to come (and as you near your baby's birth), you'll be reassured by all the tools you have to control your body's responses.

Birth is a safe and empowering experience.

ENCOURAGING ENDORPHINS

As we know, endorphins are our friend in birth and we can't produce them if we are also producing adrenaline. Start compiling a list – either an actual list or just in your mind – of your favourite songs, your favourite foods, your favourite people. These are all ideas you can draw on in labour to help generate the production of endorphins and oxytocin, which as you now know, make everything easier!

Here are my top tips for generating endorphins, keeping adrenaline firmly *out* of the equation in order to create a positive headspace:

- Find endorphin-inducing activities that you love
  This could be anything from walks in nature or watching funny movies to a romantic night in with your loved one. Schedule these things in regularly (I'm talking at least twice a week) and make them a priority. The more you practise producing endorphins, the easier and quicker it is to do.

- Talk to yourself kindly and positively
  Every morning, look in the mirror and tell yourself one thing you love about yourself. Admire your pregnant body. The voice in your head should be your biggest cheerleader. Tell yourself regularly how strong and capable you are.

- Book-end your day with calm and positive energy
  The best way to do this is to use your MP3s (see page 12). Listen to your Affirmations track in the morning when you're getting ready, and your Relaxation track as you fall asleep at night.

- Use the calm breathing technique on page 61 to stop stress in its tracks
  Whenever you feel anxious or agitated, take five calm breaths and focus on only this. Use it for anything and everything: road rage, difficult people, work situations, nerves … Using the Calm Breath in moments of stress will teach your body that this is an effective response and it will help your mind to log it as a reflex for the future, i.e. when you're in labour.

- Connect with your partner so that you feel well supported
  Read this book together, practise the face relaxation script on page 63 and soft stroking massage technique (see page 82) as often as you can, and keep the dialogue going around this exciting journey.

- Protect yourself from other people's negativity
  If someone starts to reel off their bad experience, politely tell them you'd rather pick up the conversation when you've had your own experience. And obviously don't watch reality birth programmes or films that are made for entertainment purposes.

- Focus on your own experience
  Don't worry about explaining yourself to others. It's easy for people to be sceptical or judgemental when they don't understand something, and let's face it, hypnobirthing can sound a bit 'out there' if you just go by the name. It's not your job to convince other people. This is your baby and your birth, and your energy is better spent preparing for your experience.

YOUR MIND IS A HARD DRIVE

Don't worry if you're having a tough time letting go of some of your more negative associations surrounding birth. Your subconscious mind is a bit like your own personal hard drive that you have been adding to throughout your whole life. The problem with the subconscious mind (in this instance at least) is that it can't differentiate between real information and things that we perceive to be true. It will look to store whatever it can about an event or experience without necessarily determining whether it's factual or not.

When it comes to birth, for instance, and especially when you haven't experienced it for yourself before, your subconscious mind will look for the next closest thing as a source. The media is our most common resource. This means that when we go into labour ourselves, our subconscious mind scurries through its archive and pulls up logged images of what we've seen birth is like. More often than not, these are likely to be negative impressions of birth from films and TV shows.

QUICK TIPS FOR REPROGRAMMING OUR SUBCONSCIOUS HARD DRIVE

- Start watching hypnobirthing videos (and stop watching *One Born Every Minute!*).

- Seek out positive birth stories – there are so many online and in this book.

- Ask anyone who starts telling you a negative story to wait until you've had your own experience.

- Listen to your Affirmations MP3 (see page 12) on a daily basis.

- Visualise your own positive birth – what will you be listening to? Who will be there? Engage all of your senses to create a lifelike visualisation. See page 130 for more on visualisation techniques.

- Make a vision board to represent how you want your experience of birth to look and feel. This obviously doesn't have to be images of childbirth, but sit with a few of your favourite magazines and flick through to find images you find comforting and appealing. Include images of the sea or a beach, trees, candles or soft fabrics – anything that represents tranquillity, relaxation and empowerment to you. Cut them out and stick them on a large piece of paper to look at regularly.

Where my mind leads, my body will follow.

THE MUSCLES OF BIRTH

One of the best ways to feel confident about birthing your baby is to understand exactly how your body is designed to work during labour. Think about it: if you go into labour with no concept of what your body's doing, the sensations you feel are going to be unfamiliar and possibly frightening. But if you go in understanding the functions of your birthing muscles, you'll be in a much better position to rationalise the sensations you experience and, more importantly, to work *with* them rather than *against* them.

THE UTERUS

First up is your uterus. The uterus is the female reproductive organ and it is made up of layers of strong and effective muscle (pictured opposite). Your uterus is also called your womb. It is where your baby develops until it is ready to be born. When this time comes, the muscles of the uterus work to open the cervix (the opening at the bottom of the uterus) and then push your baby down the birth path to birth. Your uterus is one amazing piece of kit, so it's important that you understand exactly what it looks like and how it works.

Essentially, your uterus looks a bit like a big balloon with an opening at the bottom (the cervix). It goes through two work phases: the opening phase and the birthing phase.

The opening phase of labour is when your cervix goes through the process of dilating from 0–10cm. For this to happen, the inner layer – made up of circular horizontal muscles – is gently pulled up by the outer layer of the uterus, which is made up of long, vertical muscles.

UTERUS MUSCLES

Outer, vertical muscles
of the uterus

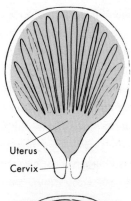

Uterus

Cervix

Middle layer of the uterus,
full of blood vessels

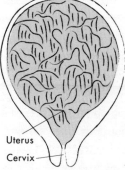

Uterus

Cervix

Inner, horizontal muscles
of the uterus

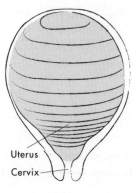

Uterus

Cervix

These muscles go up the back and over the top of the uterus, drawing up the relaxed horizontal muscles of the inner layer. The thicker muscles nearer the base of the uterus are drawn up so that the cervix slowly thins, softens and opens. These two muscle layers are designed to work in harmony, in a wave-like motion during each surge to slowly open the cervix. When your cervix is fully dilated (at 10cm), you will be ready to move into the birthing phase.

After your uterus has finished the job of opening your cervix, it nudges your baby down the birth path and some different muscles get to work. The muscle action we're talking about here is the natural expulsive reflex (NER). The natural expulsive reflex is a muscle action that is designed to expel waste from your body. The times you will be most familiar with using it are when you are sick and when you poo. Because it is a reflex, you use it without consciously controlling it. When you poo for instance, you don't need to sit down with a manual and read up on how to do it – you just get the feeling, sit on the toilet and your body does the rest. Pretty amazing really. Similarly, you'll recognise that horrible familiar feeling of wanting to be sick. You may go to bed thinking 'If I just think of something else or go to sleep, it won't happen', but of course five minutes later you have your head over the toilet because this muscle reflex has an important job to do whether you like it or not.

THE BIRTH PATH

This same muscle reflex lines your birth path (also known as your birth canal or vaginal canal). It will expel your baby from your body efficiently and comfortably. It works in a wave-like motion to rock the baby forward and back very gradually with each surge. When you birth your baby using the natural pushing action of these muscles (as opposed to forced pushing by holding your breath), your baby will be born more gently and calmly, and with a much lower likelihood of you tearing.

So, we've looked at two muscle actions here – the uterine muscle action of pulling up to thin and open the cervix, and the natural expulsive reflex muscle action of wave-like pushing to birth your baby. It is very important that you understand that these muscles are designed to work effectively and harmoniously like any other muscles in our body, but if they're going to do that, what do they need?

It's simple. All muscles need blood and oxygen to work efficiently. This is their fuel. When our muscles have a good supply of blood and oxygen, they work as they are designed to – harmoniously and comfortably. When these muscles do not have the fuel they need to work, they cannot function properly and their attempts to do so create tension and pain. Creating the optimal conditions for muscle function, with an uninterrupted supply of blood and oxygen, is key to an enjoyable birth experience. This means maintaining steady breathing throughout and allowing your body to produce the birth hormones oxytocin and endorphins by *not* producing adrenaline – i.e. it's all about remaining as relaxed and free of physical and emotional tension as possible. (See pages 146–50 for more on the hormones of birth.)

I trust my body and
follow its lead.

CHAPTER 5
LABOUR AND BIRTH

OKAY, SO THIS IS THE BIG ONE

Labour is something most women spend months and months thinking about and playing out in their minds. Where will I be? What will it feel like? How long will it last? In the event that we haven't done it before, the many unknown elements are likely to feel a bit scary at times, but it is so important to remember that labour is the completely normal and safe physiological process of bringing your baby into the world. All female mammals (well apart from monotremes, the egg-laying ones!) will labour and you and I are no different. If we can ditch the social conditioning that tricks us into thinking things are going to be unpleasant, we can consciously step aside and let our body do the work that deep down we know it is completely capable of doing.

All the strength I need is within me.

ONSET OF LABOUR

Your body is very clever and will give you plenty of signs that it is getting ready for birth. The more relaxed and in tune you are with your body, the easier they will be to recognise – so all the more reason to revisit some of those relaxation and breathing techniques and to keep listening to those MP3 downloads (see page 12).

SIGNS THAT YOUR BODY IS PREPARING FOR BIRTH:

- The bowling ball
  In the last couple of weeks of pregnancy your baby will shift down into your pelvis. On the plus side, you are likely to be able to breathe a bit easier now, as there is more space around your diaphragm and lungs, but it will also feel like you have a bowling ball between your legs! The weight of your baby's head as it engages will encourage hormones to release that will soften and shorten your cervix ready for birth.

- Putting on a show
  The release of prostaglandins will also release the mucus plug (birth show) sealing the cervix. You may not notice this, as it may just disappear down the toilet at some point, or you may see it as a blood-stained jelly-like show in your knickers. For first-time mums, labour may not begin for another couple of days but keep an eye on any cramping as this could indicate that early labour has begun.

- Waters
  Unlike in the movies, the release of the amniotic fluids is rarely a gush of water on the floor! In fact, only one in ten women will experience this before any surges begin. If you're not sure if this is happening, wear a sanitary pad for half an hour or so while you rest and if the pad is noticeably wet after this time then it is likely that your waters have indeed released. If you have released your waters, it is important to let your midwife know and note their appearance. Clear or straw-coloured and odourless is what you're looking for. There may be a slight pinky colour (remnants of the show) but green, brown or bloody or if they have a strong smell could indicate that your baby has passed meconium (their first poo) and isn't as happy as you'd like them to be.

RELAX

For most women (around 85 per cent) who do release their waters ahead of labour, surges will start within 24 hours. But it's not unusual for it to take a little longer, especially for a first-time mum. Relax while you wait and continue to monitor your baby's movements. The more relaxed you are, the more easily your body will produce those happy hormones we learned about (see pages 146–50) and the sooner your surges will begin to start labour. Also see the natural nudges on page 138.

EARLY LABOUR

The early or latent phase of labour can begin days before you are going to meet your baby. At this point, you may not even realise you're in labour, but as we've already seen, there's a lot going on behind the scenes to prepare your body and your baby for the journey ahead.

This phase of labour is often the most difficult to describe because it will vary so much between women in terms of what it feels like and how long it will last. You will be experiencing irregular surges during this time, which some women may find uncomfortable while others barely notice them. It could feel like cramping or tightening sensations. This is because your uterus is starting to warm up and surge to ease the cervix into a better position for birth. When this has happened, your surges will begin to soften, thin and open the cervix up to 3cm.

During this time, and especially if this is your first baby, it is very common to have regular surges for some hours, only for them to disappear completely a little while later. This is your body's way of taking small steps to prepare itself; one of the best things you can do during this time is to simply relax and go about your normal business. There is certainly no need to think about timing surges at this point, and your focus should be on staying relaxed and conserving your energy. If this is happening during the night, it's a really good idea to try and sleep as much as possible. Exhausting yourself now will make labour much harder further down the line, so take it as easy as possible, and start getting into your zone. Remember, this is a marathon not a sprint.

GET THOSE ENDORPHINS GOING

- Relax in a warm bath while listening to your Affirmations MP3 (see page 12).

- Get your partner to stroke or massage you (see page 82).

- Watch something funny or listen to your birth playlist.

- Maybe even get a reflexology treatment or massage (see pages 75–82).

- Remember that you want to be eating, drinking and sleeping regularly during this stage so that you have a good amount of fuel and energy on board for what's to come. Think about grazing on snacks that will tide you over and release energy slowly rather than filling you up. Smoothies, flapjacks, energy balls, nuts and dried fruit are good options.

- Going for a walk for some fresh air is a great way to get a change of scene, boost endorphins and ensure baby is in the best position for labour (see page 70 for foetal positioning).

- As you experience a surge, say the word 'open' to encourage visualisation of your cervix opening up.

- Start using the Open Breath exercise below.

In the hours or days of early labour it's advisable to stay at home as opposed to going into hospital, where it's very likely you will be sent home again. The only reasons for you to go to hospital at this point would be if your waters had released and were green, brown or black or presented a strong smell, if you are bleeding or if your baby's movements have slowed significantly. The best place for you in the latent phase of labour is at home in familiar surroundings with the person or people you love and trust.

OPEN BREATH

This amazing, expansive breathing exercise will help give your uterus the space it needs to rise and fall during labour. It will also ensure that it is fed with a brilliant supply of blood and oxygen, plus it will help you produce plenty of endorphins to boot. Use your Open Breath every single time you experience a surge, even if they are short or irregular in the beginning. Getting in the habit of doing this from the onset of labour (and even through any practice surges in the weeks leading up to the birth) means that it will be much easier to sustain when they get stronger.

1. Start by sitting comfortably and placing both feet flat on the floor. Soften your chest and shoulders so that you are holding no tension in your upper body.

2. Now imagine that there's a balloon in your tummy – give it a colour if it helps – and with your inhale imagine filling that balloon as slowly and fully as you can. When your balloon is full to capacity, I want you to exhale through the mouth, slowly releasing all of your air from the balloon. Try this now. Breathing in through your nose to fill your balloon slowly and emptying it slowly through the mouth.

3. Now try the same breath again but imagine inhaling peace and light, and exhaling any stress or tension, or if you prefer you could try inhaling a white light and exhaling a red light.

4. Another option is to inhale the word 'open' – actually visualise the word in your mind – and exhale the word 'release'.

Play around with these visualisations and see what feels good for you. There really is no right or wrong, and the reason I don't want to use a count is because every woman's breathing capacity is different, and I sometimes think introducing a count creates more stress than it resolves.

The most important thing is to pick your visualisation or technique and stick with it. Practice it every morning for five minutes when you wake up and whenever you feel stressed during the day. I guarantee if you do this, the Open Breath will become second nature, comfortable and really effective in no time at all; it will then become a trusty part of your toolkit when you're ready to bring your baby earthside.

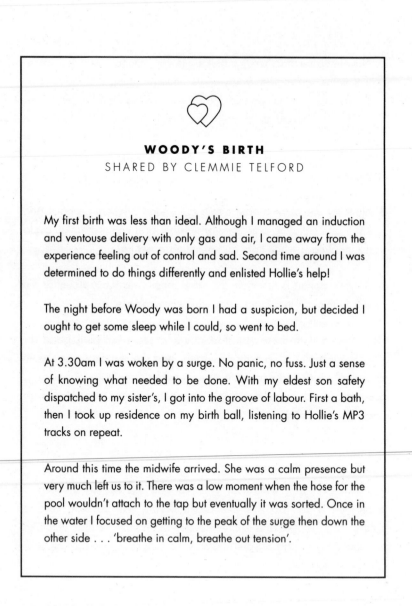

WOODY'S BIRTH
SHARED BY CLEMMIE TELFORD

My first birth was less than ideal. Although I managed an induction and ventouse delivery with only gas and air, I came away from the experience feeling out of control and sad. Second time around I was determined to do things differently and enlisted Hollie's help!

The night before Woody was born I had a suspicion, but decided I ought to get some sleep while I could, so went to bed.

At 3.30am I was woken by a surge. No panic, no fuss. Just a sense of knowing what needed to be done. With my eldest son safety dispatched to my sister's, I got into the groove of labour. First a bath, then I took up residence on my birth ball, listening to Hollie's MP3 tracks on repeat.

Around this time the midwife arrived. She was a calm presence but very much left us to it. There was a low moment when the hose for the pool wouldn't attach to the tap but eventually it was sorted. Once in the water I focused on getting to the peak of the surge then down the other side . . . 'breathe in calm, breathe out tension'.

It was hardcore. Exhausting. At the time I desperately wanted it to stop. But at no point did I feel worried or out of control. Candles, chilled music, lots of Jaffa Cakes. All very lovely.

Until transition! Suddenly the warmth of the pool felt too much. My lovely midwife suggested a change of scene. Wise move. The bright, cool bathroom felt like a new chapter.

No sooner had I taken a seat on the loo than an almighty surge hit (that's what they call 'your body taking control'). I leapt up, grabbed my husband in a strangle-hold for support and out came baby's head.

With the next surge Woody made his entrance into the world. He was born calmly and quietly with his waters intact, or 'en caul'. Swiftly followed by my placenta, which conveniently went into the toilet.

The relief was immense. I hadn't been induced. I hadn't used a scrap of pain relief. I hadn't bled. Just a tiny tear that healed naturally. I felt like the luckiest person alive!

Me and my new dude headed to bed. And that's where we stayed for the rest of the day (with Pizza Express pizza).

When people ask me about my labour, I say it was everything I wanted it to be. It was a wonderful, empowering experience, one that left me feeling that if I can breathe a baby out I CAN DO ANYTHING.

ACTIVE LABOUR

Women are often worried that they won't be able to tell when they've moved from the latent phase of labour to the active or established phase. Obviously, you won't know how dilated your cervix is, but you can trust in your ability to read the signals in your body, especially if you start listening and responding to it in this way during your pregnancy. Essentially, the main signpost of active labour is in the regularity and intensity of your surges.

The pattern that may start falling into place is around three surges in every 10 minutes, lasting at least 45 seconds each. This is known as the 3–10–45 pattern. The intensity of your surges is also likely to increase and you may need to focus more on your breath with each one at this point, which is why it's important that you get into a good breathing pattern from the onset of early labour.

When this pattern 3–10–45 happens, it's a good idea to call your midwife and let them know what's going on. Get your birth partner to do this for two reasons. The first is so that they can assert their involvement and start as they mean to go on in terms of communication, and the second is so that you can continue to relax and disengage your conscious mind as much as possible. While your midwife will want to speak to you at some point to hear how you're finding things, they can initially ask your partner questions about how you're doing and what your plan is.

If you've been having regular surges that form the 3–10–45 pattern for around two hours, you'll be assessed by a midwife if this hasn't happened already. If you are planning a home birth, your midwife will come out to your home at this point. When they arrive, they will probably just observe you for a while and have a chat with you about how you're feeling before taking some observations such as your temperature and blood pressure. They may also offer you a vaginal examination to determine how dilated your cervix is. If you are still in the latent (or 'early') phase of labour, they will leave you to relax and come back a little later, but if you are in established (or 'active') labour (3cm+) they will now stay with you until your baby is born.

If you are planning to have your baby in a hospital or birth centre, you will go to hospital for these checks. It's a really good idea to have a firm plan for getting to hospital at different times of day, and to think about having a little relaxation kit with you for the journey. This can be packed along with your birth bag, and should contain something like an eye mask, headphones (so that you can listen to your Affirmations or Relaxation MP3 track en route), a handkerchief sprinkled with some lavender essential oil and a bottle of water. Having this ready will help you to stay in your zone and make the journey less disruptive, meaning you stay in the parasympathetic nervous system (see pages 59).

When you arrive at hospital, you will go to the maternity unit reception where you will wait to be seen in triage. In triage, a midwife will take your temperature and blood pressure, and will offer you a vaginal examination to assess the stage of labour you're in. Remember that it is your choice whether or not you would like a vaginal examination. Any intervention or examination requires your informed consent, so never be afraid to say no if it doesn't feel helpful or important to you. Communicating clearly and confidently and expecting your birth partner to do the same will set the tone for the empowering and personal experience you are creating. It's worth bearing in mind that triage rooms are a stopgap and not somewhere you're going to be setting up as a nest, so take your relaxation kit in with you, keep your headphones on and let your birth partner protect and advocate for you until you can settle.

> # My surges cannot be stronger than me because they are me.

VAGINAL EXAMINATIONS

Traditionally, women are offered a vaginal examination (VE) every four hours during labour, but this doesn't mean you have to have this many, or any at all, in fact. You and your birth partner can also ask why your midwife deems it necessary at each interval, and then decide if you're happy to go ahead or not. You can also request a VE if you'd like one – some women find this useful if they're thinking about pain relief and want to know how far into active labour they are before they decide.

During a VE, your midwife will apply a sterile lubricating gel to her gloved fingers and then insert them into the vagina and upwards to feel the cervix. She is assessing for effacement and consistency of the cervix (i.e. it becoming gradually softer, shorter and thinner), dilation (between 0–10cm), whether your membranes (waters) are intact and the position and station (i.e. your baby's position in relation to your pelvis) of your baby.

Your midwife will also be observing your behaviour, sounds and even smell during labour which can help her identify the stage you are at. Remember that it's important for your birth partner to explain to your caregivers that you are practising hypnobirthing techniques, so that she can adjust her expectations accordingly. Some midwives may misjudge women who are hypnobirthing, thinking they are not as far into labour as they are because their behaviour may differ to women not using these techniques.

Other methods to tell how far along you are include looking for the purple line that will appear from the crease of your bottom and rise like a thermometer as you near completion. Your fundal height (the height of your bump while you're having a surge) can also be measured, although for this to be reliable you would need to be lying on your back during a surge, which might not be something you feel comfortable doing.

There is also a technique known as 'Mexican hot legs'. The thought behind this is that as a labouring woman's body works harder, blood is moved away from the extremities (legs) and towards the uterus (womb). This results in her legs getting gradually colder from her ankle up towards her knee as she moves deeper into labour. Normally mum's whole leg will be warm when labour begins, then around 5cm dilation the ankle to mid-calf will seem cooler, then up to the knee signals that she is moving closer to being fully dilated and ready to birth her baby.

HOW TO STAY COMFORTABLE AND RELAXED DURING A VE

- Find a comfortable position. You may need to be lying on a bed, so ask your partner to prop you up with pillows and blankets so that you're well supported.

- Remove distractions from your environment. Make sure there are no unnecessary people in the room, keep the lights dim and your birth playlist or Affirmations MP3 on. You can even slip your eye mask down to create that nice safe, dark space for yourself.

- Visualise serenity. I remember that during VEs in my labour, I would take myself off to a beach. I would close my eyes and imagine my feet being in warm, soft sand and feel gentle waves lapping across my feet. Practising this during your pregnancy will make it even easier to take yourself there during labour (see page 130 for more on visualisation techniques).

- Use your breath. Remember that calm breathing short-circuits adrenaline (see page 60) and brings about that sense of quiet stillness. Breathe in and out through your nose, trying to make the exhale longer than the inhale.

- Lean on your birth partner. Ask him or her to use the soft stroking technique (see page 82) on the inside of your arm as you breathe. This will help stimulate the production of endorphins and increase your comfort levels.

- Relax your face. Remember that tension in the jaw creates tension in the pelvis, so place your tongue behind your upper teeth and soften your mouth, or even get your birth partner to read the face relaxation script for you (see page 63).

PAIN RELIEF

Most women will want to explore their options for pain relief during labour and it is well worth talking to your midwife or caregiver about what types of pain relief will be available to you in your intended place of birth (be it home, birth centre or hospital) so that you are clear on your options and choices ahead of time. Here are the main types that you may be offered:

Gas and air

Otherwise known as Entonox, gas and air is a mixture of oxygen and nitrous oxide gas that you can breathe in through a hand-held mouthpiece. It gets to work quickly, you can control it yourself and if you don't get on with it you can just stop using it with no lasting effect. This can often work quite well for hypnobirthing mums, as it encourages you to take long, deep breaths, much like the Open Breath you've learned already (see page 166). While there are no side effects for the baby, gas and air can make some women feel sick, dizzy or light-headed, but these effects will wear off as soon as you stop using it.

Pethidine

The use of pethidine is becoming less frequent these days because of related side effects for your baby (it can affect their breathing if given too close to birth, and also their ability to feed), but it is essentially a morphine-like opioid that is given as an injection into mum's thigh or bottom during labour. It can also help you to relax. The effects of pethidine kick in after around 20 minutes and last up to four hours of the injection being administered. For this reason, it would not be given if your midwife thought you were very close to birthing your baby. Pethidine is effective in relieving pain, and will also make you feel relaxed, but it can also make you feel nauseous or 'out of it'.

Epidural

An epidural is a type of local anaesthetic (i.e. it doesn't put you to sleep) that numbs the nerves carrying pain impulses from below your waist to the brain without making you tired or sick. This type of anaesthetic will normally give you complete pain relief, although you will have very limited use of your lower body while it is in place (unless you have a mobile epidural). It can be a good option for women who have very long labours, especially if they haven't managed to sleep due to discomfort and are running out of energy. Having an epidural often means you can get some rest while your body continues to work, and you can talk to your caregivers about letting it wear off so that you still have the sensations you'll need to push if this is something you'd like to do. It's worth bearing in mind that if you have an epidural, your baby's heart rate will need to be constantly monitored so your movement may be limited, and also that it may not work straight away or require readjustment. You also wouldn't be able to use the pool or water with an epidural, as you will have a thin tube passing into your back once administered.

Spinal block

A spinal block, or 'spinal', differs from an epidural in that it delivers quick pain relief to your lower body via one injection directly into the spinal fluid (rather than in an epidural where a continuous feed of the drug is passed via a small tube threaded through the needle that goes into the epidural space). It's usually offered if your labour is progressing rapidly and delivery is likely to be soon (or in the instance of a c-section), as it requires less preparation than a full epidural and will normally only last up to two hours.

YOUR BIRTH PARTNER

Your birth partner will really come into his/her own during labour, especially with all of the wisdom and practical tools they will have picked up through practising hypnobirthing with you during your pregnancy. Their primary role is to be by your side and on your side, and there are lots of things they can be doing to help you feel comfortable, relaxed, safe and well supported. Essentially, they are protecting you from any potential distractions or stress because they are confident in their own ability to advocate on your behalf after reading a book like this. You will be approaching the birth of your baby as a team.

WAYS BIRTH PARTNERS CAN HELP DURING LABOUR:
• Remember the link between tension in your face and jaw and tension in your pelvis? If your partner can see you holding

tension in your face, they can read you the face relaxation script on page 63.

- Touch. While lots of women won't want the weight of a traditional massage during labour, there's a wonderful guide to a soft stroking technique on page 82, which helps stimulate the production of endorphins – your body's natural pain relief. It is wonderfully nurturing without being intrusive.

- Your partner can keep you comfortable with pillows, blankets, hot water bottles, fans and with helping you change position or walk around when you need or want to.

- We tend to imitate the breathing of the people around us, so here is when the breathing exercises you have practised together will come into their own. Your partner can guide you through the Calm Breath and Open Breath to keep you relaxed (see pages 60 and 166).

- Your birth partner will be the key communicator as your labour progresses. They can talk to the midwives on your behalf and then feed back information to you at a time when it's not going to disrupt your flow. They can ensure that you have the time and privacy to make informed decisions that feel right for you, and they can communicate these back to caregivers while you continue to relax.

- They can make sure you're eating and drinking regularly so that your energy doesn't fade as you progress through labour, and they can help you find more comfortable positions and keep active in the earlier stages.

- It's more than likely that you'll have lots of lucid moments in labour where you want to chat and pass the time, so your birth partner will be keeping you company here and you can enjoy these last moments of being two.

HYPNOBIRTHING YOUR WAY:

EXERCISE 10

Fun and relaxing ways to pass the time during labour:

• Listen to your favourite songs together. It's a great idea to include songs on your birth playlist that remind you of happy times in your life. Is there a song that accompanied a holiday you went on with friends or tracks from your wedding playlist, perhaps? Talk with your birth partner about what memories and feelings each song brings up for you. Reliving happy times helps generate those happy hormones that will benefit your birthing body.

• Move around. Have a dance, walk around, rock on your birth ball or lean against the wall and sway your hips. Connecting with what your body is doing and working with its movements rather than against them will help with your baby's positioning and make your labour shorter.

• Tell yourself how amazing you are. We already know that affirmations are a great way to reprogramme the subconscious mind in terms of stored beliefs (see page 86), but you can also use positive statements to boost your mood in the moment. In your head or out loud – or ask your partner to say them to you – recite 'I am strong and I am safe' or 'I'm relaxed and allowing birth to happen'. Have a look back over the other affirmations in this book too and any you wrote yourself. Mantras like this will keep you focused and keep those good hormones flowing.

• Laugh and laugh some more. A tip I often give birth partners in the run-up to labour is to keep a little log of funny things that have happened over the course of your relationship. You know those times where you feel like you are going to combust with laughter? Jot them down and relive them in labour. Laughter is one of the easiest and quickest ways to get endorphins going, so get mum's favourite funny movies or episodes downloaded for the big day too.

- Play games. Scrabble and gin rummy featured heavily during my labour! Pack some with you in your birth bag.

- Scripts and strokes. Your face relaxation script and soft stroking massage (see pages 63 and 82) should be used frequently. These are the tools that will help keep the endorphins flowing and you feeling as calm and relaxed as possible.

ESSENTIAL OILS

Essential oils are a brilliant tool for labour. Not only will they help to keep you feeling relaxed and focused, but they are also a great way for your partner to help maintain the environment and look after you.

CLARY SAGE
Diffused, inhaled or used with a carrier oil in massage, this oil has stimulating and oestrogen-regulating properties, which can boost surges as well as help ease anxiety and reduce discomfort. Do not use it before 37 weeks as it can stimulate early uterine contractions and even the onset of labour.

FRANKINCENSE
This oil can help ground you and ease any anxiety very quickly. Inhaling frankincense from a hanky can also help to regulate your breathing, so it's a nice one to combine with the Open Breath during surges (see page 166), especially if they are coming thick and fast.

JASMINE AND LAVENDER
Both of these are famously soothing and comforting. Mix with a carrier oil for your birth partner to massage into your bump or back during labour. When I was in labour, I added a few drops of lavender oil to a little face spritzer, which I found really relaxing when I was in the birth pool towards the end of my labour. Do not use jasmine oil before 37 weeks.

LEMON, MANDARIN AND ORANGE

These are great if you find you're feeling tired and sluggish and are looking for something to lift your spirits. Use in a diffuser to lift the mood of a room, especially if you've been in one place for a long time.

NEROLI AND ROSE

These are great for easing anxiety and nervousness and can help create a calming, feminine, maternal environment that makes you feel safe and centred. Definitely good ones to have on hand if you are being induced.

PEPPERMINT

A very refreshing oil that is a brilliant choice if you're feeling nauseous during labour. Rub a couple of drops on to the pulse points on your wrists and inhale from your wrists at a moment's notice.

ROMAN CHAMOMILE

A lovely addition to a relaxing set of smells, this oil can also be useful for any bruising you may experience afterwards. Adding a few drops to a bath or on to a cooled sanitary towel can help with inflammation and bruising, provided there are no open wounds.

TRANSITION

Transition is when your body has finished – or nearly finished – opening and is ready to move your baby earthside. In this moment, our primal responses kick in and we look around to check that our environment is a safe, warm and private place in which to birth our child. Because this is such a primitive time, the body releases adrenaline to put us on high alert and scour our surroundings for danger. If danger is found, we then have the power to fight off a predator, flee or freeze – to pause labour until a feeling of safety resumes. The adrenaline also gives us a second wind of energy for the birthing phase, but of course, as we have learned (see page 149), it also is likely to temporarily make the sensations of labour more powerful.

The tangible signposts of transition are often less easy to spot in hypnobirthing mums because of their high endorphin levels, which again makes it important to keep communication with your caregivers open. But at this stage, you may experience some shaking, nausea and a change in your emotional state, for example feeling overwhelmed or out of control. It's a common time for women to feel like they can't cope, that they want pain relief or even that they've had enough and want to give up.

Transition traditionally lasts 10–15 minutes, so in the grand scheme of labour it is a very short period of time, but the more understanding you have of why and what the body is doing during this stage, the more empowered you will feel in coping with it. In terms of what your birth partner can be doing here, the most important thing to offer you is a calm, secure and quiet presence.

One of the best things a woman can hear during transition, are the words: you are safe.

As soon as you feel safe, transition will pass and you will move on to the final stage. Remember, transition is a brilliant sign that your baby will be in your arms incredibly soon.

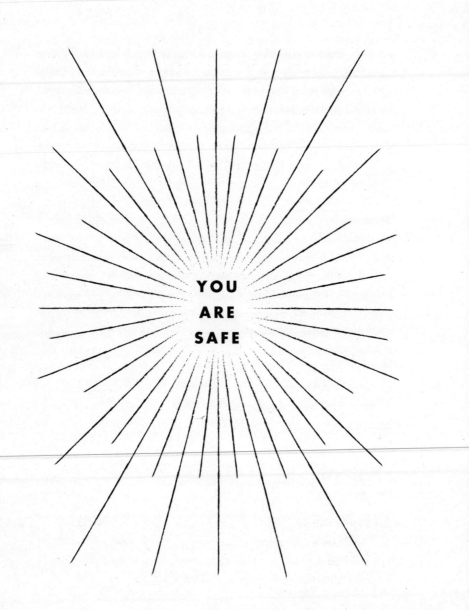

YOU
ARE
SAFE

While many birth educators don't talk about transition in any great detail, for fear of scaring women, I think it's better that you understand its place in labour so you can not only work with it when the time comes, but that it doesn't come as a shock.

TOP TIPS FOR A POSITIVE TRANSITION

• While you might feel too distracted to focus on a particular breathing technique, just try and tune into the rhythm of your own breath and visualise breathing in peace and breathing out tension.

• Find a place where you feel safe. This might be the toilet or bathroom, or in the corner of a room. Women often want to be in a dark, enclosed space during transition, so don't be afraid to follow your body's lead here.

• Make sure your birth partner knows to play your Affirmations MP3 (see page 12) at this point. Hearing these reassuring state-ments will remind you that you are safe and can do this.

• Ask for what you need. If you want to be quietly held or even left alone, don't be afraid to ask for it. Everyone is on your side and they are here to keep you safe and comfortable. Lean on them.

• Remember that you are now super close to meeting your baby, and what an exciting realisation that is. All of your hard work has paid off and you have done SO well. Your reward is within reaching distance now and you can do this.

⌐   ⌐

I know that all the sensations of birth are safe.

L   ⌐

THE FINAL PUSH

The sensation of your surges will be different now to how they felt in the opening phase of labour. Rather than the sensation of your abdominals lifting, you'll have the irresistible urge to push down. Each one of these surges, along with your natural expulsive reflex, will help guide your baby down the birth path by rocking it slowly back and forth, back and forth. It is very common to feel like you need to empty your bowels at this point and that's a really encouraging sign. The best thing to do is to sit on the toilet if it feels comfortable, as this offers a great squatting position for moving your baby down the birth path more comfortably and efficiently, and if you do need to poo then hey – you're in the right place!

The more upright you can remain during the birthing phase, the easier and more comfortable it will be for you and your baby. In this position your birth muscles will be getting the fuel they need and gravity will be on your side, too. But please note that there are really no right or wrong positions to birth your baby in. The reason I don't like being too prescriptive about what position to be in to birth your baby, is because it's important for you to tune in and respond to what your body is telling you at the time.

One of the most important things to remember here is not to hold your breath when you're pushing down. Instead, it's time for me to introduce you to the Birth Breath which will help move your baby downwards while keeping a good blood and oxygen flow to the muscles that need it.

Remember that this is just another stage of your muscles working exactly as they're meant to. Your body knows exactly how to birth your baby, and by applying your hypnobirthing rule of keeping the endorphin tap on (see pages 149–50) you'll be allowing your uterus and the muscles of your natural expulsive reflex to work efficiently and comfortably to birth your baby.

The more relaxed your body is and the more focused and quiet your mind remains, the more easily you will be able to birth your baby. Also remember that keeping a soft and relaxed jaw will have the same effect on your pelvis, allowing for your baby's easy descent. Work with your body and trust each move it makes.

BIRTH BREATH

Essentially, you are going to take a big breath in through the nose and then slowly exhale as you push – imagine taking the breath right to the back of your throat and then pushing it down through your body, guiding the way for your baby with your breath.

It can be helpful to think about the word 'down' as you breathe out, and remember only to use this breath when you're having a surge, or the irresistible urge to push.

When the surge has finished, you can quieten your mind with the Calm Breath – inhaling peace and exhaling tension, or whatever visualisation it was that worked for you (see page 130).

I want you to practise using this Birth Breath every single time you have a poo throughout your pregnancy – that way you get an opportunity to connect the breath to that expulsive reflex.

The key is to keep the breath flowing and avoid holding your breath wherever possible. If you hold your breath while you push, not only can your baby become distressed, but your natural expulsive reflex will become less efficient and you'll find yourself having to do forced pushing, which we want to try and avoid wherever possible.

As you breathe down and push with each surge, your baby will move a little further down and around the birth path. The sensation of your baby moving forwards and backwards with each surge is an entirely normal one, and a great sign that your body and baby are working together at the perfect pace.

The sensation of your baby's head pressing on the vaginal tissues and stretching the perineum sends a brilliant surge of oxytocin to the brain and this allows your baby's head to crown and be born slowly and gently.

YOU'VE DONE IT!

Once your baby's head is born, the forwards and backwards motion will subside and with the next one or two surges you will birth the shoulders and the body will slip out.

And that's it – you've done it!

You've birthed your baby and you are a goddamn goddess.

Either you or your birth partner (or your midwife if you'd like her to) will receive your baby and then put them on your chest. In the absence of any medical concerns, immediate skin-to-skin contact really is all your baby needs after birth. Your placenta is still inside you and your baby is attached via the umbilical cord, so closeness is key.

You will notice when your baby is born that the umbilical cord is still pulsating, and that's because your baby is still receiving blood from the placenta. Your baby needs this blood, so it's now advised to cut the cord only when it has stopped pulsating (see page 193 for more on this).

Your birth partner may like to cut the umbilical cord and announce the sex of your baby if you've kept it as a surprise. They will also be able to enjoy skin-to-skin with baby while you're delivering the placenta or having a shower in the hours that follow your baby's birth. Your baby will recognise your birth partner's voice if it's one they've heard regularly, so encourage your partner to talk to your bump – reading the face relaxation script on page 63 is a great place to start!

If you think about it, your baby has been as physically close to you as they can possibly be for the last nine months, so maintaining this closeness when your baby is born has a whole host of benefits for both of you. Skin-to-skin contact literally means babies being held naked against their mother (or father/other parent) and is one of the most important things you can do during the hours after birth.

BENEFITS OF SKIN-TO-SKIN CONTACT INCLUDE:

- Faster stabilisation of a newborn baby, in terms of heart and lung function, breathing and their body temperature.

- Quicker initiation of breastfeeding and stable blood sugar levels.

• A transfer of mum's good bacteria – especially important if your baby has been born by c-section and when they will have missed out on the good bacteria in the birth path and vagina.

• A calmer, more content baby because they will feel safest with the only person they've grown familiar with.

• A boost in attachment and the parent–baby bond.

THE MOMENTS AFTER BIRTH

Remember that hypnobirthing isn't just about the birth itself: it's about equipping you with the tools you need to make thoughtful and informed decisions that are in the best interest of you and your baby, in any situation. Here are some things you may want to consider on that basis for the moments after birth:

DELAYED CORD CLAMPING

This simply means not cutting the baby's umbilical cord until it has stopped pulsating, or in some cases until the placenta has been delivered. Delayed cord clamping is now becoming commonplace in UK maternity care because research has shown that its practice means babies receive 30 per cent more blood than they would with immediate clamping.

When your baby is born, the placenta will still be inside you and the baby is attached via the umbilical cord. The cord will be pulsating, which shows that your baby is still receiving oxygen, blood and nutrients from the placenta, before they finish their transactions together forever. Not only does waiting for this to happen increase your baby's blood volume, but it also increases the count of their red blood cells, stem cells and immune cells. Research also shows that keeping the cord intact immediately after birth can help prevent complications with delivering the placenta.

The World Health Organisation states that the 'optimal time to clamp the umbilical cord for all infants regardless of gestational age or fetal weight is when the circulation in the cord has ceased, and the cord is flat and pulseless (approximately three minutes or more after birth)'.

BIRTHING THE PLACENTA

A lot of women forget that once your baby is born, you still have to birth the placenta – that amazing life-giving organ that's been sustaining your baby for the last nine months. Immediately after your baby is born, it is very likely that your surges will stop, but between 10–60 minutes after the birth they will resume again, and this is so that your uterus can start expelling the placenta. For lots of women, these surges will start back up when your baby latches on to the breast and begins sucking and nuzzling, as this gives the body another surge of that wonderful oxytocin. There are two options for how to deliver your placenta, and once again, it's your job to make an informed decision of what feels right for you.

The first option is to have a physiological or natural third stage (the first stage being labour, and the second stage being the actual birth of the baby). This is when you wait for your body to start surging again, get into an upright position and expel the placenta with some gentle pushing but without any chemical interference. The only real downsides of doing it this way are that it can take a bit longer than having an 'active' or 'managed' third stage, and that there is a slightly increased risk of bleeding.

The other option is an active third stage, which is where you are given an injection of syntocinon (artificial oxytocin) which will make your uterus start surging again more quickly and help to separate the placenta from the wall of the uterus. If you do have this injection, your midwife will gently pull the cord to help deliver the placenta. This option tends to be quicker than waiting for it to happen naturally, although it can make you feel nauseous and light-headed.

Whichever way you choose to birth your placenta, your midwife will then check to see if it's intact. If you're not too squeamish, I would highly recommend having a look too, as it really is one incredible piece of kit and has done an amazing job for you and your baby.

POST-BIRTH CARE AND CHECKS
Essentially, the hours after birth are really all about bonding with your baby and lots of skin-to-skin for all of you. Your baby may be covered in vernix (the greasy white substance that protects your baby's skin in the womb). The best thing you can do is leave this to absorb into your baby's skin, and there's really no need to clean or dress them at this time.

Some babies have a bit of mucus that may need clearing from their nose and mouth and some babies need a bit of help to get their breathing established. If this is the case, your baby may be given some oxygen but they will be brought right back to you as soon as possible for lots more skin-to-skin. Your baby will then be checked over and given an AGPAR score (a measure of their physical condition including heart rate, respiratory effort, muscle tone, response to stimulation and skin coloration), but all of this can be done with your baby on you.

Whether you birth at home or in a hospital, you will be offered an injection of vitamin K for your baby. This helps to prevent a rare bleeding disorder, which your midwife should have discussed with you during pregnancy. You can opt to have this given orally instead, but they will need further doses. You can also opt out of giving it altogether.

If you do need stitches, a midwife can administer these whether you're at home or in hospital, and you will be able to carry on cuddling your baby. In the unlikely event that you have a larger tear or had an episiotomy, you will be offered a local anaesthetic for stitches or your epidural – if you had one – can just be topped up.

From here onwards, you will just continue to soak up your beautiful new bundle and enjoy the time bonding as a new family. If you're in hospital, it is likely that you'll be moved to a postnatal ward, whereas if you're in a birth centre or midwife unit you are likely to be discharged from there around six hours after the birth, all being well with you and your baby. While you're in hospital or the birth centre, try and keep your environment as calm and quiet as possible so that your baby can adjust to the world in a slow and gentle way. Keep your birth playlist on and keep the lights as dim as you are able to.

If you've had your baby at home, your midwives will stay with you for a few hours afterwards, help you freshen up and go to the toilet, and tuck you up in your own bed while they tidy up and write up their notes. Don't forget to use this time to ask your midwives any questions you have or for extra support with breastfeeding.

Never be afraid to ask for help, as there are lots of people who can help make your journey a more positive one, and it starts here.

PLACENTA CONSUMPTION

Another thing to consider ahead of time is whether you would like to keep your placenta for consumption. Stay with me.

We are one of the only mammals who don't consume their placentas after birth. Mammals consume their placentas not only to hide traces of birth from potential predators in the wild, but also because this organ contains prostaglandin and oxytocin, which both ease post-birth stress and enable the muscles around the mammaries to contract and expel milk.

In some parts of the world, women will consume their placenta either by cooking it or blending it into a paste or juice. Many of us may find it difficult to imagine wanting to do this, but placenta encapsulation (to maximise the anecdotal benefits of this practice) is becoming more and more popular.

Placenta encapsulation is the practice of turning the dehydrated, ground placenta into pills for mum to consume in the postnatal period. While little scientific research has been undertaken regarding the benefits of placenta consumption in humans, anecdotally the benefits are said to include:

- Increased release of the hormones prostaglandin and oxytocin, which help to shrink the uterus post-birth.

- Increase in the stress-reducing, corticotropin-releasing hormone (CRH).

- A reduction in post-partum depression levels and baby blues.

- A boost in iron levels in mum's blood.

- Increased milk supply.

When prepared correctly and ingested by the mother, placenta encapsulation carries no risks, which in my opinion makes it something well worth considering. If it's something you'd like to consider, I'd highly recommend having a look online at The Placenta Encapsulation Network for more information on finding a practitioner near you.

CICELY'S BIRTH
SHARED BY JULES ELVIDGE

We came to Hollie because we were given her course as a Christmas present. Neither of us really knew anything about hypnobirthing and we were both fairly sceptical; I come from a scientific background and assumed it was going to be some sort of hippie-dippy rubbish.

As the date of the course approached, I had become increasingly anxious in my pregnancy – it had started as a general underlying worry with occasional panic attacks and developed into more extreme anxiety. I couldn't sleep and I became certain I would die in childbirth. I even drafted a letter to Doug about how he should raise our unborn child without me!

Within a couple of hours on the course and Hollie explaining to us the physiology of the uterus and how birth works, I felt calm, confident and even started to feel excited about birth – it all made logical, scientific sense and she helped me to realise that my body was perfectly designed for birth and that it would be a safe and natural experience.

We threw ourselves into practising and, after a few weeks of discussion, we booked to have a homebirth and I floated through the rest of my pregnancy on a blissful cloud of calmness, confidence and excitement! We put together our birth plan but I felt fully equipped and informed to take on any turns our birthing might take.

At just over 40 weeks, in the middle of the night, my waters released gently so I got up, found a towel and went back to sleep feeling excited about what lay ahead. In the morning I woke feeling excited but had no signs of any surges starting. I called the midwife to let her know my waters had released and then went about my day doing everything I could to help my body relax and go into labour. I went for reflexology and a nice long walk and by 4pm my surges had started gently but weren't particularly regular or close together. I knew the clock was ticking and unless I was in active labour within 24 hours of my water releasing, I would have to change my plan and go to the labour ward and say goodbye to my home birth, something I desperately didn't want to do. I carefully read up on the NICE guidelines and about what my options were in this situation on the AIMS website. I felt secure that I knew what I did and didn't want, and then them focused on remaining calm and enjoying my labour.

My surges built up steadily throughout the night and when I woke in the morning they were regular and frequent. I knew I was in active labour and begged the midwife to stick to our home birth plan but unfortunately she wasn't allowed to because we'd gone past 24 hours so there was a risk of infection. So we hopped in an taxi and made our way to the labour ward.

We were met by an amazing midwife – and a rather a less-helpful obstetrician! Unfortunately, she hadn't been exposed to many hypnobirthing mothers so she refused to believe that I was in labour because I was so calm. She began (against my will) jabbing a cannula into my hands to induce me, despite my protestations and telling her that I did NOT consent. This was the moment that everything could have changed but I knew what the NICE guidance said and that she would have to listen at some point, and together with Doug and our incredible midwife, we made ourselves heard! The midwife did an internal examination to prove to her that I was in labour and found that I was 8cm dilated, so the obstetrician was sent out of the room and we were left in peace! If Hollie hadn't told us that we were entitled to refuse induction and where to find the information we needed, I know my experience would have been vastly different.

Very quickly the labour progressed and soon I was ready to breathe down our baby. It was hard work but I felt strong and my primal instincts had taken over. Within 20–30 minutes I had our beautiful baby girl in my arms. She was asleep when she came out and has remained calm and contented ever since. It was the single most incredible, empowering experience of my life.

Hypnobirthing with Hollie changed my life in a way I never could have imagined. I loved (and am loving again) my pregnancy, I had the most amazing birth, my daughter was given the best possible start to life that I could have given her, I truly am a strong, confident woman now, I am a hypnobirthing teacher myself (having been mentored by Hollie and so learned from the best!), we are expecting our second baby shortly and I am giddy with excitement about the birth and the next step in our journey.

CHAPTER 6

SO YOU'VE HAD TO THROW YOUR BIRTH PLAN OUT THE WINDOW?

HOW TO COPE WHEN SITUATIONS CHANGE

If you take one thing from this book, I hope that it's that a positive birth experience far outweighs a perfect one. Remember that I had planned a home water birth with my son and ended up with an unplanned c-section. His birth was one of the most calm and empowering days of my life because I felt fully informed and in control, even when events took unexpected turns. This was down to hypnobirthing.

You cannot predict how your baby's birth is going to unfold, but you can visualise the type of birth you want (see page 130) and equip yourself with the knowledge and techniques to navigate whatever turns it takes. Regardless of any changes in circumstances, there are plenty of ways you can make your experience a positive one. These include:

- Making sure that any suggestions for intervention are fully explained to you at all times.

- When making decisions, returning to our BRAIN acronym (see page 118).

- Maintaining an optimal environment by keeping lights dim (where appropriate), voices calm, with no unnecessary people in the room (i.e. you shouldn't feel obliged to let students observe any intervention), having your own music or MP3s playing (we had our playlist on in theatre during our c-section!) and essential oils diffusing.

- Having your birth partner with you at all times. As long as they're wearing scrubs, birth partners are generally allowed into theatre. They can be by your side keeping you calm and using the soft stroking technique (see page 82).

- Skin-to-skin contact. In the absence of your baby needing medical attention immediately after they're born, you can always have skin-to-skin contact with them, even after a c-section or instrumental delivery. If it's not possible for you to hold them, communicate that you'd like your partner to have skin-to-skin contact straight away instead. This helps enormously with regulating baby's body temperature and heartbeat, as well as with bonding (also see page 192).

- Delayed cord clamping. In the case of a c-section for example, your placenta can be removed and brought around to you in a bowl while still attached to your baby, rather than being clamped and cut straight away. This means your baby can still benefit from getting all of their blood in these moments after birth (also see page 193).

• Opting for patience over rushing. Reiterate that in the absence of a medical emergency, you're always happy to wait rather than rush the process. This removes the pressure of time protocols and gives your baby and body the space to work at their own pace.

Consider anything else that is important in making your experience a positive one and write it down. Make sure your birth partner is happy to advocate this for you in the event of circumstances changing.

I navigate my baby's birth with calmness and make informed decisions with confidence.

BETSY'S BIRTH
SHARED BY JO STAINTON

My first daughter's birth in 2012 didn't exactly go to plan. I read all the books, did NCT, talked to friends and wrote my birth plan. Not once did I prepare myself for not being in control or for an emergency caesarean. I was left pretty shell shocked and it took me a while to get my shit together.

When I discovered I was pregnant again in May 2014 all the fears I'd stuffed to the back of my mind came back to life. I felt terrified and hated the thought of going through it all again. My friend who is a midwife said she knew someone I had to meet. She introduced me to lovely Hollie and to hypnobirthing. I knew I wanted to try for a VBAC (vaginal birth after caesarean). I felt like I'd failed the first time round. Even though I'd gone through a long and hard labour, ending in a caesarean, I felt like it somehow didn't count as giving birth!

We booked on to a course in October (my EDD was early January). I thought we'd probably be experiencing a few 'and you're back in the room' moments but I was willing to give anything a shot. Right from the first session I felt differently. Hollie made us feel in control and that we had choices. We learned relaxation techniques and did breathing exercises. We discussed birth in a safe and calm environment. My husband Tom took to it immediately. There was no hippy dippy stuff, just normal people looking to learn ways to relax and welcome their babies in a calm way without fear. We watched videos of births that were so calm the babies were born asleep! We did some work on releasing fear which helped the two of us talk honestly about the things we were worried about to do with the birth. It turned out our fears were identical!

One of the fundamental things I took from the course was the belief that I had every right for my voice to be heard and that I could birth this baby the way I wanted. Over the next few weeks I began to feel really quite excited about the birth and looked forward to meeting our baby. Something I never thought I'd do.

I really wanted our daughter to enjoy Christmas without the new baby stealing the show, so I told the baby to stay put and went about enjoying our last days as a three. I'd bought a soft doll to leave for my daughter if she woke up one morning and I wasn't there because I'd gone to have the baby. I left it until the last weekend of the Christmas holidays to wrap it up and wrote her an extremely soppy card for someone to read to her. Tom said gloomily, 'looks like I'm going back to work on Monday then', and we went to bed. I felt ready.

At 4am I woke with mild pain. This time round I completely and utterly trusted my instincts: I knew this was it. I put my relaxation MP3 on and closed my eyes. I must have gone back to sleep because at 6am I woke up and realised the surges had started. I woke Tom and told him to call his parents to come and get our daughter. I got her dressed, gave her lots of hugs, packed her a bag and opened her present with her. My hormones got the better of me and I was holding back some serious tears. When she left the house at 8am the surges instantly got a whole lot stronger.

The first midwife arrived at about 10am and at that point the surges were quite strong but I was breathing through them and feeling fine. I could feel adrenaline running through me and I was trying to stay relaxed. During hypnobirthing we learnt about how adrenaline can slow labour or stop it altogether. I really didn't want that to happen.

When I was examined at 11am I was fully dilated! I couldn't believe that I'd got to 10cm without any difficulty or really any pain. Tom and the midwives started gathering towels and bin bags and began to prep our bedroom for a birth. There was a bin bag underneath me and Tom was getting ready to catch our baby! (Obviously not in the bin bag . . .) I couldn't believe I might even have a home birth!. As the surges intensified I started to push. All the while we were eating a lot of Jelly Babies (a good birth bag addition).

After a little while of pushing, time seemed to stop, as did the contractions. So I was off the bed and walking around the house, but nothing would get them going again. The longer they stopped the more anxious I became. Not because this had happened during my first birth – it hadn't – but because I could feel myself getting more and more tense and frightened that things might not go to plan.

Eventually our midwives suggested said that it might be a good idea to go into hospital to be assessed, so off we went in an ambulance; no blue lights but I felt pretty disheartened. I listened to Hollie's relaxation MP3 on my phone to drown out all the distractions.

When we got to the hospital the midwives and Tom tried to make the room as home-like as possible to make me feel calm. To my delight a scan showed the baby was perfectly positioned for a VBAC. So, with feet in stirrups, foetal monitor on and a mouth full of Jelly Babies we waited for the labour stimulating drip to kick in.

Hollie's affirmations were playing loudly the whole time and we stayed as relaxed as possible. The adrenaline was trying its hardest to take over and I was having shakes along with hysterical laughter! When the contractions started up again I couldn't feel a single one. I'd had no pain relief but I had to be told when a contraction was coming by our midwife looking at the monitor and saying 'right, go for it!', and I would focus my breath and guide the baby down. I felt like we were an amazing team, working together to help and guide me to birth the baby.

Because it was taking a while the doctor (in consultation with the midwives) decided that it might be a good idea to use a kiwi (a kind of suction cup) on the baby's head to help it down the last bit. Attaching this was possibly the only painful part of the whole labour but was over quickly.

With two big pushes the baby's head finally came out and that is when I knew we'd done it. The little body followed soon after and our midwife very quickly instructed the doctor to stand back and let Tom discover the sex and then tell me it was a little girl! Then Tom got to cut the cord. I couldn't believe it. We'd actually done it!!! And it was a girl too! I remember not quite believing what had happened.

I will never forget those moments following the birth. This little person had come from me, I felt instantly connected, instantly knowing of her. She was mine! That is what I'd missed with my first birth. Tom was so relieved everything was fine. He couldn't quite believe it either! Betsy Clementine met her big sister the following morning, and it was love at first sight.

Working with Hollie and our midwives we had managed to achieve something I never thought I would: the birth I'd wanted.

INDUCTION

Induction often feels like a big taboo that no one really understands or feels comfortable talking about, so let's take a closer look. An induced labour is one that is started artificially, and at the time of writing, around one in five labours in the UK is started this way.

At the time of writing, the most common reason for women to be induced is going overdue, however what this actually means is a bit foggy. As I've already mentioned, due dates are quite frankly something I dislike enormously, for the simple reason that they give women a completely unrealistic idea of when their baby is going to arrive. Remember that anything between 37 and 42 weeks is considered full term and is a completely normal time to have your baby, yet we are given this one date and anything either side seems to be banded as early or late – both words whose meaning can create feelings of anxiety. (See page 127 for more on estimated due dates.)

Where I live, women are routinely offered an induction at 41+3 days, so that's 10 days past their due date. Not only is this not even at the back end of full term, but it's also booked in at a woman's 40-week appointment, again setting up this idea or intention that you won't go into labour naturally, which of course has an adverse effect on how we're feeling emotionally and subconsciously at this time. Unless there's a clear medical reason for your labour to be induced, you may want to consider increased monitoring if your baby's overdue and make informed decisions day-by-day instead.

Another situation in which you may be offered an induction would be if your waters release and no surges have started within 24 hours, as the absence of amniotic fluid increases risk of infection to you and your baby. However, in some care trusts you can request antibiotics at this time, which buys you some more time for your surges to start naturally. Remember, if your waters have released, it's a great sign that your body is getting to work and labour is on its way.

Before an induction, you may also be offered a 'sweep' which can sometimes encourage labour to begin. A sweep is like a vaginal examination where your midwife will sweep their finger around your cervix in an attempt to separate the membranes from your cervix and as such kick-start your labour.

If a sweep is unsuccessful, there are two main ways of beginning the induction process. Firstly, a pessary or gel tablet can be inserted into the vagina, after which you are normally allowed to go home to wait for your surges to start.

If you aren't having surges after 24 hours, you may be offered another pessary or be invited back into hospital to start a hormone drip. The hormone drip is a synthetic form of oxytocin called syntocinon and will normally make your uterus start surging quite quickly.

A labour that has been induced in this way can often be more intense because it hasn't built up gradually like a spontaneous labour, so if you know an induction is on the cards, the best thing to do is get a really good bank of endorphins built up ahead of the planned induction, so that your body's natural pain relieving hormones are on hand to get going as soon as the surges start. (See pages 149–50.)

Being induced also does not restrict your pain relief options (see page 175) in any way, and again you can make informed decisions about what feels right for you and your baby at the time. I've said it before and I'll say it again: there is no right or wrong. This is about what feels right for you.

Before agreeing to an induction, it's important to consider that it carries its own risks. This is another reason to consider it only if there is a medical reason, rather than out of impatience.

According to NICE, between 2004 and 2005, one in five births in the UK was induced. Among these, when labour was started using drugs:

- Less than two-thirds of these women gave birth without further intervention.

- About 15 per cent had instrumental (assisted) births (such as forceps or ventouse).

- 22 per cent went on to have emergency caesarean sections.

Many women are scared about being induced, perhaps because of its medical nature, horror stories they've heard, or just the idea of things being taken out of their hands. It's really important though to remember that even if you are induced, you still have all the knowledge and tools you need to have a really enjoyable and empowering birth. Remember that it is not your uterus contracting that causes pain in labour, it's the way adrenaline inhibits the muscles' fuel supply. Keeping relaxed, calm and positive will mean you can continue to follow your body's lead and allow your muscles to work in the most harmonious way, even when they've needed a little kick-start. Practising using the tools and breathing techniques in this book will facilitate exactly that.

STALLED LABOUR

Labour is a natural process rather than a mechanical one, so it's important to remember that it's very likely that your labour and surges will ebb and flow. Sometimes, your caregivers may suggest speeding things up either by breaking your waters (if they remain intact) or with an IV drip of the induction drug syntocinon (a synthetic form of oxytocin), but before agreeing to this you should determine why it's being suggested and whether it is in your and your baby's best interest. You can use your BRAIN acronym to help you determine this (see page 118), and to find out whether induction is being suggested because you tick certain generic boxes, or because person-centred care has pointed towards a specific issue for you and your baby. Quite often in first-time mums, early labour may be long and surges may slow down or stop in order to give you a well-earned break.

If you've been awake for many hours and haven't eaten or drunk much, use this downtime as an opportunity to refuel and give your body what it needs to continue. Having a sleep in labour is not going to make things go backwards. On the contrary, women will often have a doze and then be awoken by the resurgence of their uterus getting back to work. Remember that if you and your baby are happy, there is no rush, and that the more relaxed you are, the more endorphins and oxytocin you'll be producing to aid the process of labour.

Try a change of positions or have a brief walk around – crab-walking up and down stairs is great for this – or have a little dance! I'm sure you've seen the videos online of women dancing their way through labour, and this is a great way to get gravity on your side, ease your baby down into your pelvis and trigger the flow of the hormones that help your uterus surge and cervix open.

Watch something funny to boost endorphins – now's the time to catch up on your cat videos on YouTube!

Ask your partner to give you a soft stroking massage (see page 82), have a kiss or a cuddle or even try nipple tweaking to boost oxytocin. Inhaling some clary sage oil from a handkerchief can be a good way of encouraging things along too (see pages 183–4 for more on essential oils).

Remember that your body and your baby know what to do. If you're feeling anxious, recite this to yourself out loud or in your mind, and visualise inhaling strength and exhaling fear.

My body and baby know what to do.

MY NEST IS MESSY

So what happens when your nest isn't quite as you'd envisaged it? Let's imagine you're planning a home birth but have to transfer into hospital, or the midwife looking after you isn't quite on your wavelength. What can you do to resettle in situations that disrupt your flow?

• Practise your breathing techniques as often as possible in stressful situations during your pregnancy. Using your Calm Breath (see page 60) when things don't go to plan in your everyday life will mean your subconscious logs this as an effective response to stress in the future. The more you have practised this in the run-up to your birth, the more natural it will feel to call upon it in labour, and of course the more effective it will be.

• Use essential oils at home to create anchors for relaxation (see page 183). The power of association is strong and smell is one of our most emotive senses. When you do something relaxing at home, like having a bath, going for a nap or listening to your Relaxation MP3 (see page 12), diffuse a calming oil (like lavender) at the same time. You will begin to associate this smell with being relaxed and smelling this again during labour can really help if you need a boost of tranquillity.

• Consider hiring a doula if you know in advance that your birth environment will change due to special circumstances. If a medical concern means you're going to need continual monitoring or an induction for instance, and you're going to be in a more medical environment than you'd first envisaged, you may want to look into hiring a doula who can attend your birth and help advocate for you and support you. Meet her beforehand so that you can talk about what's important to you, and as an expert in birth she will be able to help share the load with your birth partner and make sure you are getting the best care possible (see page 95 for more on doulas).

• Don't be afraid to request a different midwife. Midwives are wonderful people, but as with any area of life, there are some people whose personalities just clash with ours. Maybe you feel she isn't keen to support your wishes or has a different way of doing things to you, or maybe you just get a negative vibe from her. All of these are fine reasons for your birth partner to speak to the unit manager and ask to be looked after by someone else. There's no need to be aggressive or confrontational, it's just asking to be looked after by someone more in tune with and supportive of your needs. Remember that if you're feeling a bad energy, they probably are too, and it's much easier for you to ask for a change in midwife than for them to ask for a change in client!

• Take back-up chargers and batteries. If your labour goes on for longer than you'd envisaged or you find yourself next to noisy neighbours in hospital, the last thing you want is for your speakers or headphones to run out of charge or batteries. Make sure your birth partner has packed spares of these so that you're well equipped to relax even if you're in for the long haul.

ASSISTED DELIVERIES

Sometimes special circumstances will arise and your baby may need some help being born. An assisted birth is when forceps or a ventouse suction cup are used to help deliver the baby. In the UK, around one in eight women are currently birthing their babies with assistance, and the most common reasons for this are concerns about the baby's heart rate, the baby being malpositioned or mum being too exhausted to birth her baby on her own. Before an assisted delivery happens, your midwife will talk to you about why she thinks this is the best option and which method will be used and will ask for your consent.

If your baby is going to be born with the help of forceps or ventouse and you haven't had an epidural, you will be given a local anaesthetic to numb your vagina and perineum. This will all take place in the room you're already in in hospital, unless there are any serious concerns about the likelihood of its success, in which case you may be moved to theatre in case a c-section is necessary.

When forceps are being used, an episiotomy will be performed and then repaired with dissolvable stitches when your baby has been born. This is not always necessary with a ventouse. During each surge of your uterus, you will continue to push while your obstetrician or midwife gently pulls to help birth your baby.

When your baby is born, and in the absence of them needing medical assistance, you can still have immediate skin-to-skin (see page 192) and enjoy your baby exactly as you had intended to in your original birth preferences. Similarly, you will still have a lot of control over your environment (if you are not in theatre). Of course the lights will need to be brighter, but you can still have your own music or MP3s playing, your essential oils diffusing and your birth partner by your side to create the most calm and relaxing environment possible.

BIRTH BY CAESAREAN SECTION

Around one in five babies will be born by caesarean section. If you are having a planned c-section or a non-emergency unplanned c-section, there is a lot you can do to keep your birth preferences intact, including having your own music playing, having your birth partner with you and having immediate skin-to-skin contact when your baby is born.

A caesarean section is obviously major abdominal surgery and should only be performed if it is considered the safest birth option for you and/or your baby. Reasons for needing a surgical birth include your baby presenting in a breech or transverse position, a low-lying placenta (placenta praevia) which would obstruct the cervix for your baby's exit, pre-eclampsia, foetal distress, excessive bleeding that would put your baby at risk, or failure to progress for another reason. Some women will also choose to have a caesarean for non-medical reasons, or if they have had a previous section and don't want a VBAC (vaginal birth after caesarean).

If your baby is going to be born this way, you will be given a spinal or epidural anaesthetic. You will be completely awake for the procedure but you won't feel any pain in the numbed lower part of your body. Using your breathing and stroking massage techniques (see pages 63 and 82) can be a great way of keeping calm and grounded while your anaesthetic is being administered and you're awaiting your baby's arrival.

During the birth, which will take around 40 minutes from start to finish, a cloth screen will be placed across your body so you can't see what's being done, but you can ask for this to be lowered if you want to see what's happening – this helps some women feel more involved in the process. An incision will be made below your bikini line and you will feel some pulling/tugging as your baby is born, but this shouldn't be painful. As soon as your baby is lifted out, you and your partner will see them for the first time, and in the absence of a medical emergency, you can still do delayed cord taking by bringing the placenta around to you in a bowl with your baby for skin-to-skin. A top tip here is to put your hospital gown on back to front so that skin-to-skin is easier.

There's no reason why having a caesarean section can't be a really positive birth experience, even if it's not what you had originally planned. See the birth preferences on page 117 for more on making it as natural and positive as possible. It can also be a good idea to prepare a letter template to give to your consultant or obstetrician, in the event of an unplanned c-section:

Dear

We are using hypnobirthing techniques for the birth of our baby and would like to create a positive and empowering experience. We ask that you do your best to help us create a calm and enjoyable birth experience, even in the event of a surgical birth. We realise that because of medical reasons it is necessary to have a c-section. We request to have as natural a c-section as possible following the guidelines set out in our birth preferences, without compromising health and safety.

Yours sincerely,

BRINGING BACK THE CALM

One of the most empowering decisions you can make as you prepare for the birth of your baby is to be committed to taking control of what you can, while letting go of what you can't.

A desperation to be in control of every detail is probably going to lead to disappointment and, let's face it, is going to end the day you become a parent anyway!

Being able to adapt to changing situations in a calm way and to make informed decisions with confidence are two things you're learning to do through hypnobirthing. You are learning to understand how your mind and body work and are equipping yourself with the tools and techniques to help you during birth and beyond.

You are also learning about the power of nature, its clever intricacies and its spontaneous and changing nature.

Rather than thinking of the unknown as something scary, think of it as the magic that is yet to unfold.

Be open to following its lead and embracing the new depths of feeling it ignites within you. This is motherhood.

I take control of what I can,
and let go of what I can't.

SERAFINA'S BIRTH

SHARED BY ROXANNE HOUSHMAND-HOWELL

In March 2016 I found out I was pregnant with my second child. At our 20-week scan we were told she was a girl and that all was progressing well. After a very traumatic experience giving birth to my son – a forceps delivery followed by an emergency operation and then a blood transfusion due to severe hemorrhaging – I was anxious about having another 'natural' delivery.

My dear friend Hollie invited my husband and I to join her hypnobirthing classes. After one session I started to feel more positive about giving birth. It wasn't only her calming presence that created this sense of peace with the whole process, it was the fact that Hollie provided information about what actually is happening to our bodies during labour in a way I had never understood before. She used a different language to explain the experience, describing a contraction as a surge. This really stuck with me, the idea of surges bringing us closer to meeting our daughter.

We went away with her positive affirmations and posted them all around the home as she suggested. Each person that left our house read 'I am a strong and capable woman!' as it was stuck to the door!

At a routine appointment with the midwife, she mentioned that I was showing very big and should be tested for gestational diabetes. I wasn't too concerned and headed off to hospital for a scan and tests. The sonographer was calm and kind but I knew something was wrong as soon as she looked at the screen; her face fell and my heart sank. She quickly left the room saying she needed to find a consultant. What happened next was so traumatic that I can hardly remember much of the information given, it was just a blur of tears. Our baby girl was suffering from fetal hydrops and we were referred to Great Ormond Street Hospital for further tests. The google definition of fetal hydrops is as follows: 'fetal hydrops is not a disease, but rather a symptom of other underlying problems. It is typically triggered by chromosomal abnormalities, congenital infections, severe anemia and defects of the heart, lungs and liver. Roughly half of unborn babies diagnosed with fetal hydrops do not survive'.

At this point her chances of survival were minimal. Her body was full of fluid and her vital organs were under pressure. All I could think about was that I was now carrying a very sick baby and I felt so vulnerable and scared. I was 29 weeks pregnant and being told I had the right to terminate if I wanted to. It was a Friday afternoon and our follow-up appointment on Monday felt like a lifetime away. I spent most of the weekend crying.

But I also did what you are told not to do: I searched the internet for causes and potential outcomes. I joined the 'fetal hydrops angels' page on Facebook and prepared myself for what her death might look like. But, being optimistic, I also made a flow chart of all the potential outcomes so that I understood what my choices were and felt prepared.

On the following Monday the scan of the baby's heart and brain was positive and they couldn't detect any serious complications. However, genetic test results would take weeks and we had to be patient in trying to find the diagnosis. We decided to continue with the pregnancy. My son nicknamed our baby Sunshine.

Over the next couple of days we went straight into intensive care for an intervention to reduce the fluid so I could carry her to as near to full term as possible. I had a small operation through my tummy into the womb (the risk was that they would miss her chest wall and damage her heart) but the breathing technique that Hollie has taught us in the first session helped me to stay calm while the incredible doctors at UCLH performed their best work. A shunt was placed into my baby's chest wall to allow fluid to leave her body and take the pressure off her organs. We had scans every other day to monitor her progress.

I kept Hollie up to date with our progress. Hollie is such a calming presence and never stopped reminding me that Sunshine was a fighter and we would get through this. She sent me an MP3 for a calm caesarian – I'd lie in bed with tears in my eyes but strength in my heart that I was connected to my baby and we would get through this together. The guided meditations took me through the journey our baby and I would make.

We did really well. I managed to carry Sunshine for a further five weeks, we had frequent check-ups and monitoring while waiting for the genetic test results. They all came back negative. The doctors were still unable to diagnose the condition as we were being prepared to deliver our baby. We didn't know the outcome, how long she might survive, or what survival would look like.

On 6 January 2016 at 12.22pm Serafina Sunshine was born. We expected to spend at least a month in intensive care but Serafina was home in 48 hours. Her development was monitored for six months. Her brain, heart and lung function were all fine.

The battle was over and Serafina had won. We had all won. I couldn't have gone through it without Hollie, my family and some very dear friends.

Serafina has just had her routine developmental tests at two years old and is above average. She is very funny, very bright and beautiful.

PART THREE

AND BEYOND

Having a baby is not a series of separate events – pregnancy, birth, the postnatal period and then motherhood; it is one continuous journey. Viewing it in this way, as a whole, allows us to appreciate the equal importance of each stage and how one inevitably impacts on the others. With this in mind, we can draw on our hypnobirthing tools as we enter the sacred postnatal phase and embark on our new role as parents.

Remember that when your baby is born and for the weeks following their birth, they still believe they are part of you. They have grown inside you for nine months and it takes them many weeks after their journey to the outside world to realise that they are an independent being. It is becoming more and more common to refer to the postnatal phase as the fourth trimester and I strongly believe we should be giving it the same respect and attention as we do the stages of pregnancy and birth itself. Think of the weeks following your baby's birth day as an extension of your pregnancy and birth, an important and precious time for you to get to know this new little human and they you.

During this stage, continue to create a safe and protective environment for you and your new family – just as you did during pregnancy and birth. Take your time to adjust to this new chapter in your life. It is also important to keep talking openly with your partner, checking in with each other and asking questions. Just as when you were preparing for the birth of your baby, knowledge means you will have more choices when it comes to making decisions about how you care for your baby.

Today I will slow down and try not to rush.

CHAPTER 7
THE HOURS AND DAYS AFTER BIRTH

SKIN-TO-SKIN

You really can never have too much skin-to-skin with your baby. As noted on page 192, this precious contact encourages good attachment and bonding, can make breastfeeding easier and helps regulate your baby's heartbeat and body temperature.

The sooner you can have skin-to-skin with your baby and the more frequently you can enjoy it, the better. If for any reason you are unable to have skin-to-skin contact immediately after your baby's birth, don't underestimate the benefits of picking it back up as soon as you can. The incredible effects of skin-to-skin care extend way beyond the so-called 'magical hour' (the hour immediately following birth).

Spending as much time as possible enjoying this closeness will benefit you and your baby in the days, weeks and months to come. In fact, in the days and weeks following birth, I encourage you to be as naked as possible!

Benefits include:

- Skin-to-skin helps to regulate your baby's body temperature and helps them to feel safe and reassured as they adjust to the world.

- Breastfeeding or enjoying skin-to-skin contact while you are bottle feeding is so beneficial for your baby as it helps them to form a strong emotional attachment; partner skin-to-skin is just as beneficial here too.

- Your own body temperature increases in the weeks following your baby's birth, and this, along with night sweats (which is the body's way of expelling all of the excess fluid it stored during pregnancy) can make it feel like you constantly want a shower/ change of clothes. Keeping synthetic materials away from your skin is the best option, and what better way than to just be naked?

- Your baby can smell you and your milk, which brings them great comfort.

- You are getting used to each other and learning about each other all the time. This naked intimacy makes that so much easier and enhances emotional attachment.

FEEDING YOUR BABY

If you are planning on breastfeeding your baby, I would highly recommend learning about how breastfeeding works before your baby is born. Breastfeeding is a skill that you and your baby will learn together, and in your own unique way. It is not the same for everyone and it's important that you are able to find support if you are finding it difficult.

When I was pregnant, I remember going along to an hour's group breastfeeding class that at the time I thought was fine, but soon realised was completely inadequate. We passed around a knitted boob and looked at pictures of polar bears feeding their young. I left thinking, 'This is absolutely the best and most natural thing you can do for your baby, so how hard can it be?' I didn't leave with any information on how frequently babies need to feed, how their stomach size grows, which impacts on how often they feed and their digestive patterns, good positions for feeding, complications like tongue-tie or mastitis, or any information on mixed feeding (combining breast and bottle). The basic undertone of the class was that bottle feeding was a total last resort.

My breastfeeding journey wasn't the worst but I really didn't enjoy it. I didn't understand why my baby was feeding so frequently and felt like I'd been duped by womankind when faced with the reality of how hard it was. I became anxious every time my baby cried, for fear of him needing to feed, and this anxiety turned into tension that created pain – the very cycle I'd learned all about in hypnobirthing but couldn't connect with postnatally (see page 147).

Since becoming a hypnobirthing teacher, I've done a lot of research into breastfeeding and have worked with some incredible lactation consultants and midwives on the subject. I have learned that feeding a baby requires as much commitment and wisdom as growing one does, and that the pressure we face from our western society and the media doesn't really help or encourage women to breastfeed.

It is my belief that a positive and empowering breastfeeding journey relies on a slow and quiet immediate postnatal period. I believe that women (and their partners) need the time and space to learn about how their changing body is working, and to quietly observe how it responds to the nuances of their baby's cues. In my eyes, this has the best chance of happening in your own home, in bed, with no clothes on and no one watching you. In other words, in your nest. And it is also important to realise that this takes time.

Contrast this with the pressure women often feel to get back to their 'old selves' as soon as possible. That was so totally me. I felt like I should be out meeting friends, having coffee, going on adventures with the pram, dressing my son in all the cute onesies he'd been bought, and yet that just didn't fit with leaking boobs, raging hormones and a tiny milk monster. Next time around, I will definitely recognise that the best thing for both of us was to hole up for a bit, get a load of good box sets in, limit visitors, and get to know my baby and new body. What you lose sight of as a brand-new mum is that you have so much time to do that other stuff. Respect and cherish those early days.

Make sure you prioritise your emotional wellbeing during the postnatal period. Maybe you've already decided you'd like to bottle feed your baby, or maybe you'll decide this after your baby is born. Whatever you choose, know that if you are happy, your baby will be too. Babies primarily feed off of their mother's emotions, and making informed decisions with calmness and confidence will ensure you're giving your baby the best of you.

Today I let love lead me.

TIPS FOR A POSITIVE BREASTFEEDING JOURNEY

- Just like with birth (and with all things!), keep an open mind. Maybe even get in some bottles, a breast pump, steriliser and formula. In my experience, knowing you have options frees up your mind to make relaxed and instinctive decisions.

- Take a good breastfeeding class (personal recommendations are always best for this) and find a local lactation consultant with whom you have a good rapport. Having a chat to an expert like this beforehand will mean you feel more relaxed in seeking their support when your baby arrives.

• Find out where your local breastfeeding cafés are. Meeting other new mums who are on a similar journey to you will help you to realise that what you're feeling is totally normal and it will encourage you to ask for any help you feel you need.

• Use your hypnobirthing breathing techniques when you're breastfeeding. Before you feed, use the Calm Breath technique (see page 60) to short-circuit any fear or anxiety, and use the Open Breath (see page 166) as your baby latches on, visualising your milk flowing easily and comfortably. See also the visualisation techniques on page 130.

• Relax your mind and your muscles. You can continue listening to your MP3s (see page 12) long after your baby is born. It doesn't really matter that the content is pregnancy-focused. What matters is that it makes you feel relaxed, at ease and confident in your body's abilities. Remember the trick of putting your tongue behind your upper teeth to relax your face and jaw; this will have a positive effect on your whole body.

• Make a playlist especially for feeding. Compile a selection of songs that make you feel happy and relaxed. This will help you produce endorphins when you feed your baby and, as we know, endorphins make everything more enjoyable! The same goes for funny box sets. Laughter will get the endorphins going too! (Revisit page 148 for more on the benefits of endorphins.)

• Create a relaxing environment. Think about dim lighting, diffusing essential oils and having home comforts around you when you're feeding – many of these are the same techniques you used to create a calm environment for birth so revisit some of the ideas on pages 102–4. Lots of water and nice snacks are a must!

- Your birth partner now becomes your feeding partner! Just because you're the one with the boobs, it doesn't mean your partner is redundant. They can give you some of that lovely stroking massage (see page 82) down your arm before and/ or during a feed, or they can read the face relaxation script (see page 63) so that you feel as comfortable as possible while getting used to this new sensation.

- Sleep as much as possible during the day. Unfortunately for mums, breast milk is richer at night, plus this is when your body produces more prolactin and therefore more milk, contributing to why babies tend to feed more regularly when it's dark. Babies also can't tell day from night for the first few months of their lives, so the melatonin in your breast milk gradually helps to guide your baby into more traditional sleep cycles. Yes, I know it's hard when there seem to be so many things to do but try to sleep when your baby sleeps in the day. Definitely get it out of your head that this is in any way 'lazy' or a 'waste of time'; instead, realise that you are fuelling your tank for something awesome.

TIPS FOR POSITIVE BOTTLE FEEDING

So, what happens when breastfeeding doesn't work out, or if you'd prefer to bottle feed your baby? Remember that only you know what is best for you and your baby and that what your baby needs most is a present mother. The most important thing for your baby right now is that you feel happy and relaxed, and you should base all of your decisions going forward on this. There are lots of ways that bottle feeding can be an intimate and empowering experience for you both.

- Enjoy skin-to-skin while bottle feeding. Tucking your baby in to mimic a breastfeeding position and feeling your baby's skin next to yours while looking into their eyes as you feed them will be so wonderful and beneficial to you both. (See page 229 for more on the benefits of skin-to-skin.)

- Create a calm and relaxing environment, just as you did when you were preparing for birth. Keeping lights dim and having familiar music playing will help to remind your baby of that reassuring, womb-like environment.

- Let your partner enjoy feeding your baby too. Bottle feeding often gives mums the chance to catch up on some much-needed sleep, so definitely take advantage of this! Getting a chunk of shut-eye will mean you can be more emotionally available for your baby when you wake up.

- Remember that bottle feeding takes practice too. It may take a while to find the right bottle/teat/flow for your baby, and the best positions too, so take your time and work with your baby to establish the best feeding rituals for you.

My calmness and confidence makes my baby feel safe.

SETTLING IN AT HOME

Arriving back home with your baby, or when your midwives leave after you've had a home birth can feel super daunting. I remember arriving back home with Oscar, carrying him up the stairs in his car seat and putting him on the living room floor. His dad and I looked at each other and started nervously laughing, realising we had absolutely no idea what we were doing and were on our own with this tiny little new life! It's okay for it to feel overwhelming. Just as you did throughout your pregnancy, the more you learn about yourself and your baby as you go along, the more you are able to lean into the instinctive decisions that feel right for you and your family.

TIPS FOR SETTLING BACK INTO YOUR NEST:

- Keep lights and noises low

  Remember that your baby has been in a dark, quiet place for the last nine months. The transition to earth is a big one (for you all), so maintaining a dark, quiet environment wherever possible will help this along.

- Have a fridge/freezer full of food

  Batch cooking is a great thing to get ahead with in the days and weeks leading up to your baby's arrival – or use a meal delivery service to stock up on some hearty, nourishing meals that are going to keep you fuelled and full of energy when you need it most. Arrange for a weekly supermarket delivery so you always have the basics.

- Surround yourself with calming sounds and smells
  If you had a favourite essential oil diffusing in labour, keep it going now that you're home. Also, keep some calm or uplifting music on loop (depending on your mood). I remember having sounds of nature playing a lot of the time, which I found really comforting and relaxing, and which helped me visualise those safe places I had taken myself to in my mind during Oscar's birth.

HYPNOBIRTHING YOUR WAY:

EXERCISE 11

Although right now you're probably totally focused on the birth of your baby, make some time to really consider what your postnatal period, or the 'fourth trimester' is going to look like too. A really good exercise is to jot down some ideas of things that make you feel comforted. For instance:

- What are your favourite smells?
- What are your three most comforting meals?
- What music makes you feel happy and relaxed?
- What are your favourite magazines or books?

Once you've started to build up an idea of the things that make you feel relaxed and at ease, you can begin to get them ready for your postnatal nest. Stock up on your favourite candles and make sure you have a diffuser set up in your bedroom, as this is where you're likely to spend your first days. Remove clutter from your bedroom so that it feels like a calm space, and fill a little basket next to your bed with magazines or books that you can delve into when you're feeding or resting. Rather than giving you yet another cute outfit for your little one, ask your friends or family to cook up one of your best meals (they'll get to benefit from keeping the recipe too!) and again, start compiling a playlist that you can treasure as a soundtrack for those early days.

VISITORS

I know it's incredibly tempting in the days and weeks following your baby's birth to have all of your friends and family come and visit. Not only are they desperate to squeeze your new bundle, but no doubt you'll be super keen to show them off too! But it's really important that rather than diving straight into this, you have a think about what would really be best for you and your baby at this time.

After you've had a baby it's normal to feel a bit shell-shocked. Yes, you're going to be over the moon and in complete awe at the newest member of your family, but it's also an enormous transition. You've just discovered this huge weight of responsibility that comes with caring for this new little life. It's really normal for this to bring about a true spectrum of emotion: joy, fear, guilt, worry, pride, vulnerability and fierce protective strength to name a few.

Do you want to be riding the merry-go-round of these emotions in front of a host of visitors, or would it be better to let these feelings come and go in the safety and comfort of your own, quiet space? Often we feel like we have to put on a brave and happy face for our nearest and dearest, but I'd urge you not to do this at the expense of the emotional availability you can offer to your baby. Pleasing other people should *not* be your priority right now: looking after yourself and your baby absolutely should.

It's likely too that it will take you a good few weeks to get to grips with breastfeeding, if that's how you're choosing to feed your baby. At the beginning of this journey it's likely that you're going to take a while experimenting with positions and latch while you and your baby get used to each other, and this is MUCH easier to do without eyes coming at you from every which direction. Also, if your partner only has two weeks leave after your baby is born, then the early postnatal period becomes even more sacred. Ultimately, remember that your loved ones have plenty of time to congratulate you and admire your baby, but you and your partner will never get those first moments back.

POSTNATAL SELF-CARE

Over the past nine months or so, your body has been working incredibly hard to conceive, grow and birth your baby. Through all of your hypnobirthing practice, you've learned the importance of treating yourself kindly, listening to your body and responding to its needs. You know that when you work with your mind and body rather than against it, you'll be producing happier hormones that make everything easier and you'll be limiting anxiety and tension. This remains of paramount importance in the postnatal period too. Not only are you continuing to ride a rollercoaster of emotions mentally, but what your body has been through physically is enormous, and it's vital that you nurture it gently into motherhood.

TIPS FOR TAKING CARE OF YOURSELF PHYSICALLY AS A NEW MUM

- Get as much sleep as possible
  It sounds obvious but so many of us are conditioned to believe that sleeping during the day is lazy or indulgent. It's not. Sleep helps your body to repair and restore, and when you're up so much in the night, it's essential that you're catching up on this magic ingredient during the day. In fact, you should be prioritising it above anything else. To-do lists and tidying can wait.

- Book a postnatal massage or therapeutic treatment
  Again, I really consider this to be an essential, rather than a luxury. If you think about what your body has achieved physically, it's important that you help to restore and realign it in the weeks after birth. A good postnatal massage can help to alleviate tension in the body, especially in the upper back and shoulders, which can be brought on by breastfeeding. Massage also helps circulation and boosts lymphatic drainage as your body starts to expel all of the excess fluids from pregnancy, and it promotes sleep by relaxing your mind and muscles. Remember that when we relax we produce those wonderful endorphins that make the world

seem like an easier place! You could also look into therapies such as reflexology, osteopathy and acupuncture to help with physical realignment post-birth. (See pages 72–84 for more on the benefits of massage and other alternative therapies.)

- Move your body gently
  A postnatal exercise routine is probably the last thing on your mind, but starting to move and stretch your body *gently* will get those endorphins going and help you get back in touch with yourself physically. Rather than diving into anything too strenuous, go for a short walk around your local park or even just around the block, using your Calm Breath technique (see pages 60–61) as you walk. Don't walk quickly, just be mindful of your steps and become aware of your body's movements and your breath. You could also do a short postnatal yoga routine. There are some great apps that allow you to do a virtual class at home. Start with something very gentle for 15 minutes and build this up only when you feel ready. If you've had a c-section, I'd highly recommend booking a post-caesarean Pilates course. This is brilliant for helping to heal the body after a surgical birth and slowly build abdominal strength again in a safe way. Make sure to check with your caregiver that you are ready. You can also pick up the pelvic floor exercise we looked at on page 53, and again, anchor it into an activity you're doing regularly so that you don't forget to do it.

- Book a pedicure or blow-dry
  I know this one sounds silly and overly girly, but it's amazing what a tiny bit of pampering can do for your mood and the way you feel about yourself physically. A few weeks after you've had your baby, book an appointment for a pedicure or haircut.

Both of these won't inhibit you holding your baby and you'll be free to feed or cuddle them while you're being looked after. You'll feel like a new woman on the other side.

⌐   ⌐

I love, nurture and enjoy my amazing body.

L   J

TIPS FOR TAKING CARE OF YOURSELF EMOTIONALLY POSTNATALLY

- Focus on your breath

  Our breath is our greatest tool. I know you already know that through doing all of the hypnobirthing breathing techniques during your pregnancy and birth, but the benefits don't stop here! Start every day with five minutes of that wonderful expansive Open Breath (see page 166) to fill your system with oxygen and give yourself an immediate boost. Before each feed, use your Calm Breath (see page 60) to diffuse any tension or anxiety, and do the same after a feed too.

- Surround yourself with nourishing smells
  Just like you did during your pregnancy and labour, you can use reassuring and comforting smells to calm your senses or boost your mood. Diffuse natural essential oils around your house or burn your favourite scented candle. This is the time to indulge and nurture.

- Listen to your MP3s or a relaxing playlist
  Keep your Affirmations and Relaxation MP3s playing (see page 12). The content may not be as relevant now, but they will anchor you back into the relaxation you felt during your pregnancy and birth. Or invest in one of our postnatal MP3s (see www.londonhypnobirthing.co.uk/shop) for motherhood or breastfeeding to take with you on your journey.

- Hire a postnatal doula
  Sometimes you could just do with a bit of help and, if finances allow, a doula can assist you however you need them to in the postnatal period – they can do a bit of cleaning or cooking or generally just look after you. This can really ease the pressure off a new mum's shoulders and help her to rest and look after her baby without trying to juggle everything else.

- Talk it out
  Remember that it's good to talk, especially when you're experiencing such a range of emotions postnatally. Don't be afraid to ask for help from friends, your GP or your midwife and express how you're really feeling. If you've had a difficult birth or feel like you are struggling to cope postnatally, make an appointment with a therapist or counsellor who can help you to explore your feelings in a safe and nurturing way.

- Put yourself first

  Don't feel like you have to please everyone all of the time. If you've had a bad night with baby and are feeling exhausted and emotional, take the day off and just lie in bed with your baby and Netflix! Feed, snooze, read, breathe – do whatever your mind and body need on a daily basis and don't plan too far ahead. Taking each day as it comes is the key to a happy postnatal period.

CHAPTER 8
I AM A GREAT MOTHER

ONWARDS AND UPWARDS

So here we are at the end of one journey and of course, at the beginning of another. Much of the practice of hypnobirthing is attributed to its power during the birth of your child, but hopefully you can see now that it offers so much more than that. Hypnobirthing has given me some of my most valuable life tools, from trusting my body; learning how to make informed decisions and being more confident in asking questions around my own wellbeing; and to leaning into my instinct and intuition when I haven't always made a habit of doing so in the past. Hypnobirthing has also empowered me with the mindset that everything is temporary, a lesson that has served me well – and continues to – in my life as a mother. With adaptable and simple tools and techniques that help you to short-circuit stress and return to a place of calm, you can trust that you are more than well equipped to navigate this journey, one day at a time.

That said, motherhood is challenging, tiring and confusing at the best of times, so don't put too much pressure on yourself to breeze through it like a maternal goddess. You are learning all the time and so is your baby. The physical and emotional rollercoaster of motherhood is something that everyone experiences differently, and something you will deal with best if you feel well rested and nurtured and take your time to find your way. This, of course, is easier said than done, but I'm going to try and break it down into my top tips for protecting your emotional wellbeing and enjoying the ride. Here goes.

COMPARISON IS THE THIEF OF JOY

Remember that just as with everything in life, people do things differently. What works for one rarely works for another, and we're all trying to find that bit of equilibrium where things feel right for us. This will depend on all sorts of things – your beliefs and values, finances, career, relationships, culture – and one of the best pieces of advice I can offer is to focus on your own journey. Use your hypnobirthing wisdom to tune into your intuition and gut instinct, just like you did during your pregnancy, and apply it now that your family has grown. Also, don't compare yourself to strangers on the internet (or even your own friends). Social media can be a wonderful thing, but remember it's just people showing the highlights of their lives and hiding away the washing-up pile, the dirty pants and the arguments about whose turn it is to take the bins out. Let the online world connect and inspire you, but take it with a pinch of salt in terms of reality.

YOU DO YOU

Remember that BRAIN acronym (see page 118) we learned earlier in the book? It applies now too! Whenever you need to make a decision, either as a mother or on behalf of your child, go through those questions to reach an informed choice. Knowing the benefits, risks and alternatives of all of your options (and of course applying the instinct/nothing rule) GIVES you options. You can apply this to lots of things – feeding, vaccinating and healthcare, childcare, parenting styles, schooling – the list really does go on. If you feel uncomfortable with other people's opinions, remember that you don't have to tell everyone what you are or aren't doing, and you certainly don't need to explain your choices to others. This is your journey and nobody else's, so you do you, proudly and confidently.

THIS TOO SHALL PASS

Try to remember that everything is temporary; you have survived everything that life has thrown at you so far, and will continue to do so. Sleep deprivation certainly led me to catastrophise the most basic of problems, and actually it wasn't until I leaned back into my relaxation and breathing techniques that I was able to snap out of this habit. You will have days where you are exhausted and feel unable to function. Your baby will have days where they are fractious and unsettled. On these days, do what you have to do to get through. If that means going for a long walk with the buggy and some headphones, or getting a friend or relative over to sit with your baby while you have a bath or a nap, or even just cancelling plans and hanging out on the sofa in your pyjamas all day – DO IT! It's okay to put yourself first and to prioritise your emotional wellbeing right now. Cancelling plans is okay, especially if it means you're saving your energy for your baby and yourself.

FIND YOUR TRIBE

Don't feel like you have to be friends with people just because they had babies at the same time as you. You are a woman with an identity, and you are just as capable now as you've always been of forging friendships with people who make you feel loved, make you laugh and are compassionate towards you. If people aren't floating your boat or are draining your energy, move towards people who do the opposite. You are no less of a woman now that you're a mother, and you have so much to offer your baby AND the world. I've made lifelong friends through becoming a mother, and finding people who you can be honest and vulnerable with, as well as have a laugh and a glass of wine with, is invaluable! Pick your dream team, just like you did when you were preparing for the birth of your little one.

CELEBRATE THE VICTORIES AND ACKNOWLEDGE THE CHALLENGES

Despite my best-laid plans for a beautifully scripted, emotive journal of my first few months of motherhood, I was definitely way too tired to write much sense. However, at the end of each day I would just jot down what I'd achieved that day (FYI, I still never write to-do lists, but *always* do a 'ta-dah' list – writing down what I've achieved at the end of the day is so much more rewarding!) and also what I'd found really hard. I remember in the early days my partner getting home and asking what we'd been up to (in a caring way) and feeling bad at not being able to think of anything substantial enough to mention. This is a rubbish feeling, but the truth is we do SO much as mums that goes unseen. When I started writing my ta-dah list and acknowledging how many small achievements I'd made, it really shifted my sense of productivity and pride. And yes, making a sandwich or washing your hair goes on the list! In terms of writing down what's been challenging, this is really helpful too because it gives you a healthier perspective on everything you're navigating on a daily basis – much of it completely new territory. Balancing these lists at the end of the day will definitely help you reflect on just how brilliantly you are doing.

Lastly, I'd really like to encourage you to be kind to yourself, and bring your thoughts back to the exercise on page 48, where you gave advice to a friend who's going through something difficult. Try it again now when you're feeling overwhelmed or anxious, because it really does work. Write down how you're feeling and what has made you feel that way, and then imagine replying as a friend with some words of comfort and compassion.

This is your time and you are well equipped to give your baby everything he or she needs, simply by being you. You do enough, you have enough and you are enough, and mama – you always will be.

I am exactly what my child needs.

A FINAL WORD

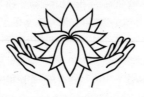

As a woman, you are fully equipped to bring your baby into the world in a safe and empowered way. With the hypnobirthing practice you are prepared to put in, you will be able to draw upon all of your skills and trust in the power of your baby and your body during pregnancy and birth – and beyond.

You have a system in place that is perfectly designed to work efficiently and powerfully. It is your job to remove anything that may be holding you back in your mind and that may be inhibiting your body from performing in these amazing ways. Give lots of time and thought to the type of birth experience you want. Talk to your birth partner every day about what you can be doing together to prepare for meeting your child, and work to become a solid and loving team during labour.

Your body really does know what to do. Your focus now is to release all limiting thoughts and fears around birth so that you aren't hijacked by them when your body begins to labour. Producing adrenaline inhibits your birthing muscles from working comfortably and effectively, so every single day I want you to practise the visualisation and breathing techniques I've given you to short-circuit that stressor response in your day-to-day life. The more you get used to using this, the more it becomes an instinctive response for your mind and body in times of stress, and the more easily you will be able to switch off your conscious mind in labour and go within to harness your inner strength.

Remember to create a team of people around you who are supporting you in your choices. If you're not happy with something, speak up. Don't be afraid to ask questions and request the kind of care that makes you feel nurtured and empowered.

I cannot stress enough that practice is key. You will get as much out of this book as you put into it, so please give it the same weight as you would any other important commitment in your life.

Remember, too, that your baby's birth is one day alone. Their experience starts now, in your belly, and continues through to the moment you are holding them in your arms and beyond as you become a family. Hypnobirthing is about approaching this experience in a holistic way. It is a journey and it is here to be lived and enjoyed in a way that is personal to you. If you practise daily, it will become such a normal and instinctive part of your life. When you feel more in tune with your own emotional beliefs and how you feel physically, you will make day-to-day decisions based on how you truly feel. This will help you to have an empowering experience of life as a person and as a parent. With your partner supporting you in this, you become the ultimate team and a strong, loving family unit develops. This is what the world needs, and it starts with you.

I'm going to leave you now with some words by my heroine, Ina May Gaskin. Ina May Gaskin has been described as 'the mother of authentic midwifery' and I highly recommend checking out anything she's written.

We are the only species of mammal that doubt our ability to give birth. It is profitable to scare women about birth but let's stop it. Giving birth can be the most empowering experience of a lifetime – an initiation into a new dimension of mind-body awareness. Wherever and whenever you intend to give birth, your experience will impact your emotions, your mind, your body and your spirit for the rest of your life. So even if it has not been your habit throughout life so far, I recommend that you learn to think positively about your body.

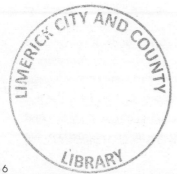

ACKNOWLEDGEMENTS

I cannot quite believe that I have actually written this book. There are some very special people who have helped this dream of mine to become a reality, and it really wouldn't exist without them.

First, I want to thank Sam Jackson for convincing me that this book was inside me. Your belief in me from the beginning has been unwavering and your constant support and encouragement is the reason *Your Baby, Your Birth* exists. I'd like to extend this appreciation to the whole team at Penguin Random House and Vermilion: to my editors, Leah Feltham, Laura Herring, Anne Rieley and Clare Sayer, whose attention to detail is magnificent, and to publicity and marketing gurus, Sarah Bennie and Rebecca Hibbert, for having such a brilliant vision for my voice and beliefs. Thank you to Emma Scott-Child and Zoë King at Junction Studio for bringing to life how this book looked in my mind (and for drawing and re-drawing endless amounts of vaginas), and to Philippa James who somehow managed to photograph me looking half-reasonable when I was in the depths of morning sickness! You are all true professionals and getting to work with people who are as good at their jobs as you guys are makes me feel very lucky.

Thank you to Jessica Stone and Alistair Skeoch, my agents at Independent Talent Group. You have this beautiful way of making my life about 150 times easier and I appreciate everything you've done to support this project and me as a person.

Your Baby, Your Birth is what it is because of the voices of wisdom and comfort scattered across its pages and I feel very privileged for it to feature some of the best in the baby business: Hannah Adams,

Claire DaBreo, Beccy Hands, Nancy Nunn, MaryAnne Shiozawa, I'm looking at you here. I'd like to extend this gratitude to the other birth professionals I've been lucky enough to work with: Gemma Connell, Jules Elvidge, Sam Hazelgrove, Laura Jones and Imogen Unger. The women of London are lucky to have you guys working among them because you work in an empowering and nurturing way that really changes lives. Thanks, also, to my own hypnobirthing teacher, Sophie Birch.

Thank you to every woman who has shared her birth story with the readers of *Your Baby, Your Birth* and inspired other women to value their own capabilities. Thank you to Fearne Cotton, Giovanna Fletcher, Izzy Judd and Russell Brand for supporting this book and my vision with your kind and positive words.

To the talented people behind the scenes at yesmum HQ – Carly Hardman and my mum, Sally, without whom my business wouldn't function – and to the personal and professional mentors who have always cheered me on and given me a nudge in the right direction when I needed it; Steve Ball, Roxanne Houshmand, Helen Lang, and Tayo Popoola, you are four of life's gems. To the friends who have kept me sane and smiling while writing this book and when life has thrown its curveballs. You know who you are and I love and appreciate you.

It might seem strange to thank your ex-husband in your acknowledgements but, Christian, I would never have even gone to that hypnobirthing class if it wasn't for you. Oscar's birth really was the highlight of my life and I will never forget it, or the profound role you played. You are the most wonderful father to our boy, and always have been, and I feel lucky to parent alongside you.

Next, I really want to thank my precious family. Thanks to my grandparents, Mama and Gandy, and to my mum and dad for instilling the kind of work ethic inside me that I have learned (painfully at times) one can't write a book without. You have always provided me with so much love and it wouldn't be mine to share if it wasn't for you. You've always supported me even when you haven't agreed with my choices, and that is what I appreciate the most. Also to Jack, Laura and Archie – I love you very much.

Thank you, Simon, for coming into my life exactly when you were meant to. You make me believe in the magic of timing and of love. Thank you for telling me otherwise when I thought I couldn't write this book, for your unfaltering belief in my abilities and for always, always, making me feel incredible. My life is better with you and Manolo in it, and I can't wait for the next part of our adventure to begin. Our family may not be conventional, but it will always be full of love. You are one of life's good ones. Don't change.

Finally, to Oscar. You, my darling boy, started it all. The day I became your mother was the day I realised I could do anything. You have changed me so profoundly and you remind me every day what really matters. You are kind and compassionate, you are funny and smart and you are a loving human being. Every day you make me proud, and being your mama is the biggest honour of all. I love you, and this book is for you.

INDEX